English - Chinese
Chinese - English
Nuclear Security Glossary

Committee on the U.S. - Chinese Glossary of Nuclear Security Terms

Committee on International Security and Arms Control
Policy and Global Affairs Division
U.S. NATIONAL ACADEMY OF SCIENCES
THE NATIONAL ACADEMIES

Chinese Scientists Group on Arms Control
CHINESE PEOPLE'S ASSOCIATION FOR
PEACE AND DISARMAMENT

THE NATIONAL ACADEMIES PRESS
Washington, D.C.
www.nap.edu

ATOMIC ENERGY PRESS
Beijing
www.aep.com.cn

National Academies Press

The National Academies Press was established in the early 1980s as the official publisher of the National Academy of Sciences, the National Academy of Engineering, the Institute of Medicine, and the National Research Council. NAP employs approximately 75 people and has 10 departments: Administration, Composition and Graphics, Design, Editorial, Digital Strategies, Fulfillment and Warehouse, Marketing, Printing, Production, and Reprographics.

The project that is the subject of this report was approved by the Governing Board of the National Research Council, whose members are drawn from the councils of the National Academy of Sciences, the National Academy of Engineering, and the Institute of Medicine. The members of the committee responsible for the report were chosen for their special competences and with regard for appropriate balance.

This study was supported by Contract No. DE-AT01-06NA26358, TO #16 between the National Academy of Sciences and the U.S. Department of Energy. Any opinions, findings, conclusions, or recommendations expressed in this publication are those of the author(s) and do not necessarily reflect the views of the organizations or agencies that provided support for the project.

International Standard Book Number-13: 978-0-309-11931-3

International Standard Book Number-10: 0-309-11931-6

Additional copies of this report are available from the National Academies Press, 500 Fifth Street, N.W., Lockbox285, Washington, D.C. 20055; (800) 624-6242 or (202) 334-3313 (in the United States); Internet, http://www.nap.edu

Atomic Energy Press

The Atomic Energy Press (AEP), established in 1973, is a national specialized publishing house. It grew out of the former Editorial Board of Nuclear Science Committee of Chinese Academy of Sciences, which was established in 1959. The AEP, subordinated to the China National Nuclear Corporation (CNNC), edits and publishes scientific and technical books, textbooks, periodicals and dictionaries in the nuclear field, and books and reference works in relevant fields.

※ ※

图书在版编目(CIP)数据

汉英/英汉核安全术语/中国人民争取和平与裁军协会，
美国国家科学院编著. —北京：原子能出版社，2008.4
ISBN 978-7-5022-4102-5

Ⅰ. 汉… Ⅱ. ①中…②美… Ⅲ. 核工程-安全技术-术
语-英、汉 Ⅳ.TL7-64

中国版本图书馆 CIP 数据核字 (2008) 第 038028 号

汉英/英汉核安全术语

出版发行	原子能出版社 (北京市海淀区阜成路 43 号　100037)
责任编辑	卫广刚　李代斌
印　　刷	绵阳市科学城曙光印刷厂
经　　销	全国新华书店
开　　本	787mm×1092mm　1/16
印　　张	17
字　　数	420 千字
版　　次	2008 年 4 月第 1 版　2008 年 4 月第 1 次印刷
书　　号	ISBN 978-7-5022-4102-5
印　　数	1—2000
定　　价	128.00 元

COMMITTEE ON THE U.S. - CHINESE GLOSSARY OF NUCLEAR SECURITY TERMS

CISAC GLOSSARY TEAM

Chair

Ming-Shih Lu Ph.D., Brookhaven National Laboratory (retired)

Members

Richard L. Garwin Ph.D., Thomas J. Watson Research Center, IBM Corporation (emeritus)

Raymond Jeanloz Ph.D., University of California, Berkeley

Alastair Iain Johnston Ph.D., Harvard University

Alvin W. Trivelpiece Ph.D., Oak Ridge National Laboratory (retired)

Staff

Benjamin J. Rusek Senior Program Associate, Committee on International Security and Arms Control

Anne Harrington Director, Committee on International Security and Arms Control

CSGAC GLOSSARY TEAM

Chair

Tian Dongfeng Ph.D., China Academy of Engineering Physics

Members

Hu Side Member of the Chinese Academy of Engineering, China Academy of Engineering Physics

Zhu Jiaheng Beijing Institute of Applied Physics and Computational Mathematics

Shi Jianbin Beijing Institute of Applied Physics and Computational Mathematics

Wu Jun Ph.D., Beijing Institute of Applied Physics and Computational Mathematics

Yu Xiaoling Chinese Scientists Group on Arms Control

He Yidan Chinese Scientists Group on Arms Control

Kang Chunmei China Academy of Engineering Physics

Sun Xiangli Ph.D., Beijing Institute of Applied Physics and Computational Mathematics

Tian Jingmei Ph.D., Beijing Institute of Applied Physics and Computational Mathematics

THE NATIONAL ACADEMIES

Advisers to the Nation on Science, Engineering, and Medicine

The National Academy of Sciences is a private, nonprofit, self-perpetuating society of distinguished scholars engaged in scientific and engineering research, dedicated to the furtherance of science and technology and to their use for the general welfare. Upon the authority of the charter granted to it by the Congress in 1863, the Academy has a mandate that requires it to advise the federal government on scientific and technical matters. Dr. Ralph J. Cicerone is president of the National Academy of Sciences.

The National Academy of Engineering was established in 1964, under the charter of the National Academy of Sciences, as a parallel organization of outstanding engineers. It is autonomous in its administration and in the selection of its members, sharing with the National Academy of Sciences the responsibility for advising the federal government. The National Academy of Engineering also sponsors engineering programs aimed at meeting national needs, encourages education and research, and recognizes the superior achievements of engineers. Dr. Charles M. Vest is president of the National Academy of Engineering.

The Institute of Medicine was established in 1970 by the National Academy of Sciences to secure the services of eminent members of appropriate professions in the examination of policy matters pertaining to the health of the public. The Institute acts under the responsibility given to the National Academy of Sciences by its congressional charter to be an adviser to the federal government and, upon its own initiative, to identify issues of medical care, research, and education. Dr. Harvey V. Fineberg is president of the Institute of Medicine.

The National Research Council was organized by the National Academy of Sciences in 1916 to associate the broad community of science and technology with the Academy's purposes of furthering knowledge and advising the federal government. Functioning in accordance with general policies determined by the Academy, the Council has become the principal operating agency of both the National Academy of Sciences and the National Academy of Engineering in providing services to the government, the public, and the scientific and engineering communities. The Council is administered jointly by both Academies and the Institute of Medicine. Dr. Ralph J. Cicerone and Dr. Charles M. Vest are chair and vice chair, respectively, of the National Research Council.

www.national-academies.org

THE CHINESE PEOPLE'S ASSOCIATION FOR PEACE AND DISARMAMENT

Founded in June 1985 by various concerned non-official organizations and prominent personages from all walks of life in China, the Chinese People's Association for Peace and Disarmament (CPAPD) is the largest nationwide non-governmental peace association with a total of 24 important member organizations.

The objectives of the CPAPD are to promote mutual understanding, friendship and cooperation between the peoples of China and the rest of the world in joint efforts to maintain world peace, oppose arms races and war, achieve arms control and disarmament, strive for the complete prohibition and thorough destruction of nuclear weapons and other weapons of mass destruction, protect ecological environment and promote economic development and social progress.

Having established a wide range of friendly contacts and ties abroad, the CPAPD undertakes cooperation and exchanges in various forms with more than 300 NGOs and research institutions in about 90 countries, which work for peace and conduct research in the fields of arms control, disarmament, global or regional security.

While actively engaged in research on such issues as arms control, disarmament, peace and security, the CPAPD sponsors or co-sponsors various academic seminars annually, sends scholars and experts to attend international conferences or seminars, and hosts visiting delegations from abroad.

The CPAPD has Consultative Status with the Economic and Social Council (ECOSOC) of the United Nations and is a member of the Conference of NGOs (CONGO) in Consultative Relationship with the United Nations.

ACKNOWLEDGMENTS

The glossary committee members and staff have benefited greatly from the insights and observations of well-informed officials and scientific colleagues in the United States and China. The views that were obtained during these discussions were essential in providing a basis for the glossary. The committee expresses its gratitude for the time that these colleagues devoted to helping ensure that this glossary is as complete and accurate as possible.

The glossary has also benefited from previous work by a number of organizations, both U.S. and Chinese. In particular, we would like to acknowledge the Nuclear Threat Initiative and the Monterey Institute on International Studies for allowing us to access work they did in 2002 on a nuclear terms dictionary. We also would like to acknowledge the Editing Committee of the *National Defense Science and Technology Dictionary-Nuclear Energy Column*, the Editing Committee of the *Arms Control and Disarmament Handbook*, and the Editing Committee of the *Chinese Military Encyclopedia*. Many terms and definitions in the glossary are quoted from their achievements.

This glossary has been reviewed in draft form by individuals chosen for their diverse perspectives and technical expertise in accordance with procedures approved by the National Research Council's Report Review Committee and by the joint Review Committee organized by the Atomic Energy Press and the Chinese People's Association for Peace and Disarmament. The purpose of these independent reviews is to provide candid and critical comments that assist the institutions in making this published glossary as sound as possible and ensure that the glossary meets institutional standards for objectivity and accuracy. During the review, comments and the draft manuscript remained confidential to protect the integrity of the process. We wish to thank the following individuals for their review of this report:

U.S. Reviewers

Ping Lee	National Security Technologies, LLC, Division Leader
Stephanie Lieggi	Monterey Institute of International Studies, Research Associate
James Mulvenon	Center for Intelligence Research and Analysis, Director, Defense Group Inc.
Brad Roberts	Institute for Defense Analysis, Research Staff
Christopher Twomey	Naval Postgraduate School, Assistant Professor and Associate Chair for Research
Jing-dong Yuan	Monterey Institute of International Studies, Director, East Asia Nonproliferation Program

Chinese Reviewers

Qian Shaojun	Member of the Chinese Academy of Engineering, PLA General Armament Department, Senior Researcher
LiMin	Member of the Chinese Academy of Sciences, Beijing Institute of System Engineering, Senior Researcher
Song Jiashu	Member of the Chinese Academy of Sciences, China Academy of Engineering Physics, Senior Researcher
Zhu Xuhui	China National Nuclear Industry Corporation, Senior Researcher
Yan Shuheng	China National Nuclear Industry Corporation, Senior Researcher
Liu Gongliang	Beijing Institute of Applied Physics and Computational Mathematics, Senior Researcher
Niu Qiang	Chinese People's Association for Peace and Disarmament, Secretary-general
Duan Zhanyuan	The Department of Defense, Senior Researcher
Ouyang Liping	China Institute of Contemporary International Relations, Senior Researcher
Wei Guanggang	Atomic Energy Press, Editor

Although the reviewers listed above have provided many constructive comments and suggestions, they were not asked to endorse the publication, nor did they see the final draft of the glossary before its release. The review of this report was overseen by R. Stephen Berry, the University of Chicago. Appointed by the National Academies, he was responsible for making certain that an independent examination of this publication was carried out in accordance with institutional procedures and that all review comments were carefully considered. Correspondingly, in China the review was finally supervised by Qian Shaojun, Member of the Chinese Academy of Engineering. He was elected by the review committee members and led the committee to examine and verify the terms thoroughly, especially the terms with definition. Responsibility for the final content of this report, including its objectivity and accuracy, rests entirely with the authoring committees and institutions.

PREFACE

The Chinese Scientists Group on Arms Control (CSGAC) of the Chinese People's Association for Peace and Disarmament, and the Committee on International Security and Arms Control (CISAC) of the U.S. National Academy of Sciences have been meeting for almost 20 years to discuss nuclear arms control, nuclear nonproliferation, nuclear energy, and regional security issues, with the goal of reducing the possibility of nuclear weapons use and reducing nuclear proliferation in the world at large.

Throughout these rich exchanges, our discussions have benefited from the contribution of bilingual participants and the services of interpreters. Despite long-standing personal relationships and strongly shared interests between CSGAC and CISAC, it was often evident that beyond the never-simple translation of one language into the other, there was also the difficulty of differing interpretations of terms.

With substantial and growing international efforts in nonproliferation of nuclear weapons, counter-proliferation and the prevention of nuclear terrorism, and with the expansion of the use of nuclear power and the role of international inspections, it is important that participants whose respective native languages are Chinese and English agree on the meanings given to relevant terms in the two languages. In cases where they cannot agree, then it is important that they understand the usage in the other language, and be aware that a simple statement of the term may have alternative or ambiguous meanings.

In April 2006, CISAC and CSGAC considered a joint project to produce an unclassified glossary of nuclear security terms, and concluded that this was feasible and would be valuable. Accordingly, participants on the two sides formed working groups and developed a framework for the glossary, and CSGAC prepared an initial set of terms. The working group members used e-mail intensively during this development phase, and also held joint meetings in Beijing in September 2006 and again in March 2007. Following several more rounds of e-mail consultations, the text was reviewed in China and the United States by experts from both countries whose comments and clarifications are reflected in the final manuscript. CISAC and CSGAC finalized the list of terms, definitions, and references at a November 2007 joint working group meeting. We believe that the product of this project, a joint CISAC and CSGAC glossary, will be a valuable resource to the government, academic, and security community.

This glossary of approximately 1000 terms is intended to reduce the likelihood of misunderstanding, and to remove barriers to progress in exchanges and diplomatic, cooperative, or other activities where unambiguous understanding is essential. For many of the terms, this is just a matter of translation because, in our review, we could readily agree on an appropriate translation of the term volunteered by one side or the other. Consequently, there was little likelihood of misunderstanding, and so the majority of the terms in this glossary are simply paired with the corresponding term in the other language.

Another category of terms required definition. It was clear that although there might be a single meaning in one language, there were several possible options that dealt with matters that were quite distinct in the other, For these terms, we have arrived at what we believe to be a common definition, which, in turn, we present in both languages.

A third category of terms is one in which there are different meanings even within a single language. That is, the same set of words is used in different contexts to describe different objects, actions or concepts. For these terms, although we have in many cases agreed on a single translation of the term, we felt it necessary to provide varying interpretations that might be encountered for example, in military or diplomatic circles.

Where possible, we have taken our definitions from reputable preexisting sources in authoritative texts or preexisting glossary compilations. We have given preference to international documents, then to official governmental documents, and then to organizations or references of some standing such as the National Academy of Sciences, the *Arms Control and Disarmament Handbook* (军备控制与裁军手册), the *National Defense Science and Technology Dictionary-Nuclear Energy* (国防科技名词大典——核能卷), and similar sources. We have published the work as a book in the conventional Chinese-English and English-Chinese format. In addition, we have published the same source material on the Internet in a more "user friendly" format at:
http://www8.nationalacademies.org/webglossary and at:
http://www.cpapd.org.cn/webglossary.

Because terminology continues to evolve, we expect that an expanded version of the physical book may be produced at some future point. It is our intent to update the on-line version routinely, as the scope of interaction increases and clarifications come to light. We have arranged to do this in a transparent fashion; on-line one can see the changes and updates as well as the original version.

The committees intend to formally review the list of terms approximately one year following publication and will make additions and corrections as needed at that time. The committees welcome comments on the glossary at: cisac@nas.edu and at: css@iapcm.ac.cm

P

Finally, we would like to especially thank Dr. Richard Garwin of CISAC and Academician Hu Side of CSGAC for providing invaluable guidance during all phases of this project. We are very proud to have had their participation as the U.S. and Chinese committee leaders and technical guides for the preparation of this glossary.

Ming-Shih Lu Dongfeng Tian

April, 2008

CONTENTS

GLOSSARY ORGANIZATION AND CONTENT

I Glossary Organization

This glossary is divided into English and Chinese sections. In the English section, terms are arranged in alphabetical order, while in the Chinese section, terms are arranged in the order of *Pinyin* (Chinese phonetic alphabet). Each page has two columns, one in English and one in Chinese. In the Chinese section of the glossary, the Chinese column is on the left, while the English column is on the right. In the English section, English is on the left and Chinese is on the right.

In the Chinese section, which is arranged in the order of *pinyin*, for those terms whose first characters' *pinyin* are the same, they will be arranged in the order of Chinese tones: high and level tone (the first tone, i.e. ā), rising tone (the second tone, i.e. á), falling-rising tone (the third tone, i.e. ǎ), and falling tone (the fourth tone, i.e. à). If the *pinyin* and the tones are all the same, terms will be arranged by the number and sequence of the strokes of the Chinese characters. If every aspect of the first character is the same, the rule applies to the consecutive characters of the term.

The English section is arranged in alphabetical order without regard to capitalization.

For convenience of reference, terms are also classified by category. There is a categorization index before the main glossary section. The first level indicates the broad category, the second level index indicates the subfield under the category, and the third level index indicates the specific term. In the Chinese section, the index is in Chinese, while in the English section, the index is in English. Numbers following the terms indicate the page location in the corresponding language section. For example:

NUCLEAR ARMS

Nuclear Weapon

strategic nuclear weapon·················70

tactical nuclear weapon··················73

II Glossary Content

The information provided in the glossary generally consists of the term in English, Chinese, and *pinyin* and for defined terms a definition, and/or source, note, or reference. The definitions for the selected terms are only given in English and Chinese, not *pinyin*. Other terms also include expanded information in both Chinese and English, depending on the need for clarification of use, sources, and other considerations.

A Terms

Terms generally are words or phrases (with *pinyin* following the Chinese term). For example:

nuclear weapon 核武器【héwǔqì】

The use of parentheses - ( ) - in a term indicates that the words in parentheses can be used as 1. another way of expressing the term 2. notes related to the term or 3. an abbreviation. For example:

1 nuclear underground (or underwater) burst
2 DUPIC (Direct Use of Spent PWR fuel in CANDU reactors) process
3 command, control, communication and intelligence system (C3I)

A symbol like "/" in the term's name means the word(s) before and after "/" have the same meaning. For example:

diversion strategy / diversion path

B Pinyin

Every character in a term's Chinese name is marked with its *pinyin* according to the standard Chinese pronunciation system. Chinese *pinyin* words are separated from each other by a blank space. For example:

战略核武器【zhànlüè héwǔqì】

Characters in the neutral tone are only marked with their phonetic alphabets without tones. For example:

保障监督的质量保证【bǎozhàng jiāndū de zhìliàng

bǎozhèng】

If a character in a term is not Chinese, it will be directly used in the term's *pinyin*. For example:

无源 γ 射线探测 【wúyuán γ shèxiàn tàncè】

Punctuation marks in terms' names are omitted in their *pinyin*. For example:

发方/收方差额 【fāfāng shōufāng chā'é】

C Definitions and sources

The name of the term is generally not repeated in its definition. The glossary provides at least one source for each defined term, but cites only the source passages containing the definition. If a term's definition is identical with that in the source, the definition will be noted as "From:"; if term's definition is modified using the source, it will be noted as "Modified from:" If a term has two or more definitions, the glossary lists those definitions and sources separately.

The terms' definitions include a sequence number for the sources and the source page numbers where appropriate. With the sequence number, detailed information on the source can be found in the "References" section of the glossary.

D Notes

If a term's content needs an additional explanation, the glossary adds "note". For example:

tag

……

Note: An active tag requires electrical power, while a passive tag works without a power supply.

E Cross-reference

If one term's content relates to others, the glossary adds "Refer to". For example:

core of atomic bomb

Refer to "**pit**"

III References

This section contains detailed information on the sources quoted in the glossary. The references are listed in Chinese and English, are formatted for ease of comprehension in both English and Chinese and include the maximum amount of information available to assist the reader locate the original source. In general the references are ordered by author(s), title, and if available publication location, publisher, publication date, date of last on-line access, and on-line address. Additional information such as the edition, volume, or document number is included for some references. Since several references are cited more than once, references page numbers are included with the definition in the body of the glossary text.

IV Other Information

The "*General List of Simplified Chinese Characters*" as published by the National Language Working Committee, October, 1986 serves as the standard for all Chinese characters in this glossary. The "*National Standard of People's Republic of China" GB/T 15834—1995* serves as the standard for all Chinese punctuation marks in the glossary. The "*National Standard of People's Republic of China" GB/T 15835—1995* serves as the standard for all numbers in the glossary. But all numbers have not been separated by commas. The "*National Standard of People's Republic of China" GB 3100～3102—93* serves as the standard for all Chinese units of measurement or science and technology marks in the glossary. The Chinese text of the glossary generally uses Arabic numerals, except for those numbers which are commonly expressed in Chinese numerals in China.

INDEX

(in alphabetical order)

PART 1 ARMS CONTROL AND DISARMAMENT

1 Arms Control, Disarmament and International Security

2 International Law for Arms Control and Disarmament

3 Geneva and United Nations' Main Disarmament Organizations

4 Treaties, Agreements Related to Nuclear Arms Control and Disarmament

PART 2 NUCLEAR ARMS

1 Nuclear Strategy

2 Nuclear Weapon

3 Delivery/Launch System of Nuclear Weapon

PART 3 NUCLEAR TEST BAN

1 Treaty Banning Nuclear Weapon Tests

2 Nuclear Test and Monitoring

PART 4 PROHIBITION OF THE PRODUCTION OF FISSILE MATERIAL FOR NUCLEAR WEAPONS

1 Legal Instruments and Other Documents Related to

IAEA Safeguards

2 IAEA Safeguards

3 Nuclear and Non-Nuclear Material

4 Nuclear and Nuclear-Related Activities and Installations

5 Nuclear Material Accounting

6 Nuclear Material Verification and Monitoring

PART 5 NON-PROLIFERATION

PART 6 CONFIDENCE BUILDING MEASURES

PART 7 VERIFICATION OF ARMS CONTROL AND DISARMAMENT TREATIES

PART 8 BASIS OF NUCLEAR SCIENCE

absorbed dose	吸收剂量【xīshōu jìliàng】
absorption	吸收【xīshōu】
Accelerated Strategic Computing Initiative (ASCI) Note: The program has been changed to Advanced Simulation and Computing Program (ASC). (From: Reference [37])	加速战略计算倡议 【jiāsù zhànlüè jìsuàn chàngyì】 注：现已改为“先进模拟与计算计划”。(源自：参考文献[37])
account balance	账面平衡【zhàngmiàn pínghéng】
accounting records	衡算记录【héngsuàn jìlù】
acquisition strategy/acquisition path A (hypothetical) scheme which a State could consider to acquire nuclear material usable for manufacturing a nuclear explosive device. (From: Reference [4], 3.8)	采办策略/采办途径 【cǎibàn cèlüè cǎibàn tújìng】 某国谋取用于制造核爆炸装置的核材料的一种(设想)策略。(源自：参考文献[4]，3.8)
active defense Note 1: A term used to describe China's military strategy. It includes the following main elements: firstly, taking a firm stand of self-defense and gaining mastery by striking only after the enemy has struck; secondly, using active military preparations and political struggle to prevent war; thirdly, should war break out, using active counter-attack and offensive operations to achieve strategic defensive objectives. (Modified from: Reference [31], p124-125) Note 2: In the U.S., "active defense" is the employment of limited offensive action and counterattacks to deny a contested area or position to the enemy. (From: Reference [9], p4) Note 3: In the context of missile defense, "active defense" means the	积极防御【jījí fángyù】 注 1：用以描述中国军事战略的术语。它主要包括以下三方面的内容：一是坚持自卫立场和实行后发制人；二是以积极主动的军事准备和政治斗争防止战争；三是一旦战争爆发，以积极的反击和进攻作战达成战略防御目的。(改自：参考文献[31]，p124-125) 注 2：在美国，“积极防御”指采取有限的攻击及反击以防止敌方占领竞争中的区域或地点。(源自：参考文献[9]，p4) 注 3：在导弹防御领域，“积极防御”指拦截并摧毁导弹或其弹头；

E-C

interception and destruction of missiles or their warheads; "passive defense" is protection against the effects of the warheads primarily by the use of blast shelters, stockpiling of food, etc. (Modified from: Reference [62])	"消极防御"指主要通过使用爆炸掩体和食物存储等来抵御弹头的效用。(改自：参考文献[62])
active neutron detection A method of determining the existence of fissionable material through detecting the neutrons emitted from the fission that is induced by an external source. (From: Reference [1], p495)	有源中子探测 【yǒuyuán zhōngzǐ tàncè】 利用外源诱发裂变材料裂变，通过探测裂变发出的中子而证实裂变材料存在的方法。(源自：参考文献[1], p495)
active nuclear stockpile	现役核武库【xiànyì héwǔkù】
active seal Refer to "**seal**"	有源封记【yǒuyuán fēngjì】 参见"封记"
active tag Refer to "**tag**"	有源标签【yǒuyuán biāoqiān】 参见"标签"
active warhead	现役弹头【xiànyì dàntóu】
Ad Hoc Committee of Conference on Disarmament	裁军谈判会议特设委员会【cáijūn tánpàn huìyì tèshè wěiyuánhuì】
ad hoc inspection	特别视察【tèbié shìchá】
Additional Protocol	附加议定书【fùjiā yìdìngshū】
aftershock detection	余震监测【yúzhèn jiāncè】
Agreed Framework Between the United States of American and the Democratic People's Republic of Korea	美朝框架协议 【měi cháo kuàngjià xiéyì】
agreement	协定/协议【xiédìng xiéyì】
Agreement Between the United States of America and the Union of Soviet Socialist Republics on the Establishment of Nuclear Risk Reduction Centers	美苏关于建立减少核危险中心的协定 【měi sū guānyú jiànlì jiǎnshǎo héwēixiǎn zhōngxīn de xiédìng】

Agreement Between the United States of America and the Union of Soviet Socialist Republics on the Prevention of Nuclear War	美苏关于防止核战争协定【měi sū guānyú fángzhǐ hézhànzhēng xiédìng】
Agreement on Measures to Reduce the Risk of Outbreak of Nuclear War Between the United States of America and the Union of Soviet Socialist Republics	美苏关于减少爆发核战争危险的措施的协定【měi sū guānyú jiǎnshǎo bàofā hézhànzhēng wēixiǎn de cuòshī de xiédìng】
Agreement on the Privileges and Immunities of the IAEA	国际原子能机构特权和豁免协定【guójì yuánzǐnéng jīgòu tèquán hé huòmiǎn xiédìng】
alarm system for physical protection	实体(实物)保护报警系统【shítǐ shíwù bǎohù bàojǐng xìtǒng】
alert rate of nuclear missiles The percentage of those missiles that are on various stages of alert and can launch in stipulated preparatory times in relation to the entire arsenal of deployed missiles. (Modified from: Reference [2], p49)	核导弹的戒备率【hédǎodàn de jièbèilǜ】 处于各种戒备状态并能在规定发射准备时间内实施作战发射的导弹数占部署导弹总数的百分比。(改自：参考文献[2]，p49)
ammonium diuranate	重铀酸铵【zhòngyóusuān'ān】
announcement	公告【gōnggào】
annual dose	年(辐照)剂量【nián fúzhào jìliàng】
annual throughput	年通过量【nián tōngguòliàng】
anti-ballistic-missile missile	反弹道导弹的导弹【fǎndàndàodǎodàn de dǎodàn】
anti-coercion alarm Also called anti-hijack alarm. The concealed warning device provided for guards on duty or on patrol. (Modified from: Reference [2], p91)	反胁迫报警【fǎnxiépò bàojǐng】 又称反劫持报警。给值班、巡逻人员配备的隐蔽报警装置。(改自：参考文献[2]，p91)
aquafluor process	水氟化流程【shuǐfúhuà liúchéng】

aqueous reprocessing	水法后处理【shuǐfǎ hòuchǔlǐ】
area target	面目标【miàn mùbiāo】
arming nuclear weapon	核武器解保【héwǔqì jiěbǎo】
arms control	军备控制【jūnbèi kòngzhì】
arms race stability	军备竞赛稳定性 【jūnbèi jìngsài wěndìngxìng】
artificial radionuclide	人工放射性核素 【réngōng fàngshèxìng hésù】
ASEAN (Association of Southeast Asian Nations) Regional Forum	东盟地区论坛 【dōngméng dìqū lùntán】
assassin's mace A type of metal weapon. Chinese classical novels describe the means of throwing the mace at the adversary unexpectedly in order to win during fighting. It is a metaphor for an adept ability or unique skill used at a critical moment. (Modified from: Reference [36])	杀手锏【shāshǒujiǎn】 锏是一种由金属制成的冷兵器。在中国古典小说中指与敌厮杀时出其不意地用锏投掷敌手、以求取胜的招数。喻指在关键时刻使出的最拿手的本领或称绝招。(改自：参考文献[36])
asymmetric warfare A war in which either side employs a different weapon, tactic or strategy. "All strategy works on asymmetries, so asymmetric warfare is representative of all rationally executed warfare." (From: Reference [55], p102-108)	非对称战争【fēiduìchèn zhànzhēng】 任何一方使用了不同的武器、战术或战略的战争。"所有战略都基于非对称性原则进行谋划和实施，因此理性运筹的战争都具有非对称性特征。"(源自：参考文献[55]，p102-108)
atmospheric nuclear test	大气层核试验【dàqìcéng héshìyàn】
atmospheric-pressure fuze of nuclear weapon	核武器气压引信【héwǔqì qìyā yǐnxìn】
atomic bomb	原子弹【yuánzǐdàn】
Atomic Energy Commission	原子能委员会 【yuánzǐnéng wěiyuánhuì】

atomic mass	原子量【yuánzǐliàng】
atomic nucleus	原子核【yuánzǐhé】
atomic number	原子序数【yuánzǐ xùshù】
atomic-vapor laser isotope separation	原子蒸气激光同位素分离法【yuánzǐ zhēngqì jīguāng tóngwèisù fēnlífǎ】
attribute approach Identifies treaty-limited objects by measuring certain characteristics of an object that should be displayed by all items of a given general type. (Modified from: Reference [11], p104)	属性法【shǔxìngfǎ】 通过测量物项的某些特征来识别条约限定物项的方法。这些特征为某特定类型的所有物项所具备。(改自：参考文献[11]，p104)
attributes test A statistical test of a characteristic (or attribute) of an item to which the response is either "yes" or "no". (From: Reference [4], 10.30)	属性检验【shǔxìng jiǎnyàn】 判断一个物项的某项特征(或属性)为"是"或"否"的统计试验。(源自：参考文献[4]，10.30)
authentication	真实性验证【zhēnshíxìng yànzhèng】
ballistic-missile early warning system	弹道导弹预警系统【dàndàodǎodàn yùjǐng xìtǒng】
ballistic-missile submarine	弹道导弹潜艇【dàndàodǎodàn qiántǐng】
ban	禁止【jìnzhǐ】
baseline data inspection	基准数据视察【jīzhǔn shùjù shìchá】
baseline exhibition for non-nuclear heavy bombers	非核重型轰炸机基线展示【fēihé zhòngxíng hōngzhàjī jīxiàn zhǎnshì】
batch data	批数据【pīshùjù】
beginning inventory of nuclear material The amount of nuclear material at the beginning of a balancing period. It should be equal to the inventory at the	核材料初期存量【hécáiliào chūqī cúnliàng】 某一衡算周期开始时所拥有的材料量。初始实物存量应等于前次材料衡算周期中核材料的末期存量。(源

E
I
C

end of the last material balancing period. (From: Reference [2], p186)	自：参考文献[2]，p186)
bilateral cooperation agreement	双边合作协定【shuāngbiān hézuò xiédìng】
binding energy	结合能【jiéhé'néng】
boiling water reactor (BWR)	沸水堆【fèishuǐduī】
book inventory of a material balance area	材料平衡区的账面存量【cáiliào pínghéngqū de zhàngmiàn cúnliàng】
boosted atomic bomb	助爆型原子弹【zhùbàoxíng yuánzǐdàn】
burnup	燃耗【ránhào】
calibration	校准【jiàozhǔn】
canned subassembly (CSA) The secondary assembly in a nuclear weapon containing both fusion fuel and in most cases uranium (some or all of which may be HEU). (From: Reference [11], p90) Note: In America, the subassembly that is to be incorporated into the final weapon is called a "canned subassembly"	罐装组件【guànzhuāng zǔjiàn】 核武器的次级装置，其内包含聚变燃料和(大多数情况下)铀装料(可能部分或全部是高浓铀)。(源自：参考文献[11]，p90) 注：在美国，要装入最终武器的部件被称为"罐装组件"。
capability of destroying hardened target	毁伤硬目标能力【huǐshāng yìngmùbiāo nénglì】
capability of destroying soft target	毁伤软目标能力【huǐshāng ruǎnmùbiāo nénglì】
cascade	级联【jílián】
centrifuge damping device	离心机阻尼装置【líxīnjī zǔní zhuāngzhì】
centrifuge failure rate	离心机失效率【líxīnjī shīxiàolǜ】
centrifuge rotor dynamics	离心机转子动力学【líxīnjī zhuànzǐ dònglìxué】

centrifuge rotor material	离心机转子材料 【líxīnjī zhuànzǐ cáiliào】
centrifuge separation plant	离心分离工厂【líxīn fēnlí gōngchǎng】
chain reaction	链式反应【liànshì fǎnyìng】
charter	宪章【xiànzhāng】
China's nonproliferation export control system China's comprehensive export control system regarding various nuclear, biological, chemical and missile-related sensitive items, technology and all military goods.(From: Reference [38])	中国防扩散出口管制体系 【zhōngguó fángkuòsàn chūkǒu guǎnzhì tǐxì】 中国关于核、生物、化学和导弹等各类敏感物项和技术及所有军品的全面的出口控制体制。(源自：参考文献[38])
circular error probable (CEP) For repeated trials, the radius of a circle enclosing half of the impacts of a projectile, missile, or bomb. (Modified from: Reference [9])	圆概率偏差【yuán gàilǜ piānchā】 对于射弹、导弹或炸弹而言，其圆概率偏差是指，在反复试验中，包含其半数弹着点的圆形区域的半径。(改自：参考文献[9])
classical super design	经典超级模型 【jīngdiǎn chāojí móxíng】
classification of reactor	反应堆分类【fǎnyìngduī fēnlèi】
clean hydrogen bomb	干净氢弹【gānjìng qīngdàn】
close-out inspection	设施关闭视察 【shèshī guānbì shìchá】
closed-down facility/closed-down location outside facilities	已关闭设施/已关闭的设施外场所 【yǐguānbì shèshī yǐguānbì de shèshīwài chǎngsuǒ】
closed nuclear fuel cycle There are two common types of nuclear fuel cycle. One is the "open" fuel cycle, in which the spent fuel is not reprocessed but kept in storage pending eventual disposal as waste. The other is the "closed" fuel cycle, where the spent fuel is reprocessed and the uranium and plutonium separated from the fission	闭式核燃料循环 【bìshì héránliào xúnhuán】 核燃料循环通常有两种类型。一种是"开式"燃料循环，即乏燃料不经过后处理，在最终处置前以废料形式储存。另一种是"闭式"燃料循环，即乏燃料经过后处理从裂变产物中分离出铀和钚。铀和钚都可

products. Both the uranium and the plutonium can be recycled into new fuel elements. (From: Reference [14], p1-2)	作为新的燃料元件循环使用。(源自：参考文献[14]，p1-2)
cobalt bomb Refer to "**induced-radioactivity bomb** "	钴弹【gǔdàn】 参见“感生放射性弹”
cold war	冷战【lěngzhàn】
collective radiation dose	集体辐照剂量【jítǐ fúzhào jìliàng】
collective security An approach to prevent and curb aggression and maintain security for countries through the organized collective action of multiple countries. (From: Reference [1], p23)	集体安全【jítǐ ānquán】 多国通过有组织的集体行动来预防和制止侵略，保护各国安全的一种方式。(源自：参考文献[1]，p23)
command, control,communication and intelligence system (C3I)	指挥、控制、通信和情报系统(C3I 系统) 【zhǐhuī kòngzhì tōngxìn hé qíngbào xìtǒng C3I xìtǒng】
command, control,communications, computing and intelligence (C4I)	指挥、控制、通信、计算和情报系统(C4I 系统) 【zhǐhuī kòngzhì tōngxìn jìsuàn hé qíngbào xìtǒng C4I xìtǒng】
Committee on Disarmament	裁军谈判委员会 【cáijūn tánpàn wěiyuánhuì】
common security A security concept that originated in Europe during the Cold War era. In 1982, the Independent Commission on Disarmament and Security Issues chaired by Swedish prime minister Olof Palme published a report entitled "Common Security: A Blueprint for Existence", which for the first time put forward this concept. The report pointed out that common security is based on the following concept: the best guarantee for security is obtained through cooperation in improving	共同安全【gòngtóng ānquán】 冷战时期欧洲形成的一种安全概念。1982 年，瑞典首相帕尔梅主持的“裁军和安全问题独立委员会”的报告《共同安全：生存蓝图》中首次提出。该报告认为，共同安全是基于这样一种认识，即安全的最佳保证是通过双边或多边的增强安全合作而非通过相互竞争的强权政治来获得。(源自：参考文献[1]，p23)

security for both or all parties rather than through competitive power politics.(From: Reference [1], p23)	
communication system for physical protection	实体保护通信系统 【shítǐ bǎohù tōngxìn xìtǒng】
communique	公报【gōngbào】
compellence The use of the threat of force to compel a desired action by one's adversary. (From: Reference [23]) Note: compellence refers to efforts to stop an action already underway whereas deterrence refers to efforts to prevent future action. (From: Reference [39]) Derived from: "Compellence… usually involves initiating an action (or an irrevocable commitment to action) that can cease, or become harmless, only if the opponent responds." (From: Reference [23])	威逼【wēibī】 威胁使用武力以迫使敌手采取己方期望的行动。(源自：参考文献[23]) 注：威逼致力于终止已发生的行为而威慑致力于防止未发生的行动。(源自：参考文献[39]) 衍生：威逼，通常包括发起(威胁性)的行动(或诉诸行动的不可更改的决心)，只有在对手作出(妥协性的)反应后才能终止或变得无害。(源自：参考文献[23])
complex (diffusion) barrier A kind of (isotope) separation barrier composed of multiple layers of compactly overlapped porous barriers with different structure. (From: Reference [2], p81)	多层分离膜/复合分离膜 【duōcéng fēnlímó fùhé fēnlímó】 由多层不同结构的多孔膜紧密叠合组成的分离膜。(源自：参考文献[2], p81)
composite sample	混合样品【hùnhé yàngpǐn】
comprehensive (full scope) safeguards agreement (CSA)	全面保障监督协定 【quánmiàn bǎozhàng jiāndū xiédìng】
comprehensive national power	综合国力【zōnghé guólì】
Comprehensive Test Ban Treaty (CTBT)	全面禁止核试验条约 【quánmiàn jìnzhǐ héshìyàn tiáoyuē】
compressor for gaseous diffusion separation	气体扩散分离压缩机 【qìtǐ kuòsàn fēnlí yāsuōjī】

computer simulation of a nuclear explosion	核爆炸的计算机模拟【hébàozhà de jìsuànjī mónǐ】
concert of powers	大国协调【dàguó xiétiáo】
Conference of the Committee on Disarmament (CCD)	裁军委员会会议【cáijūn wěiyuánhuì huìyì】
Conference on Disarmament (CD)	裁军谈判会议【cáijūn tánpàn huìyì】
Confidence and Security Building Measures (CSBMs)	建立信任与安全措施【jiànlì xìnrèn yǔ ānquán cuòshī】
configuration of hydrogen bomb	氢弹构形【qīngdàn gòuxíng】
contact fuze of nuclear weapon	核武器触发引信【héwǔqì chùfā yǐnxìn】
containment of nuclear material	核材料封隔【hécáiliào fēnggé】
containment strategy Refers to the foreign policy strategy of the United States during the Cold War in which it attempted to stop the expansion of the Soviet Union and to prevent nations moving politically towards communism led by the Soviet Union. (Modified from: Reference [40])	遏制战略【èzhì zhànlüè】美国在冷战初期试图阻止苏联的扩张和防止一些国家在政治上走向苏联领导的共产主义的外交政策战略。(改自：参考文献[40])
continental shelf	大陆架【dàlùjià】
continuous inspection An inspection regime intended to maintain continuity of knowledge concerning inventory and flow of nuclear material by witnessing key operations, recording measurement and operating data, and verifying the information in order to meet the safeguards objectives. (From: Reference [4], 11.12)	连续视察【liánxù shìchá】为达到保障监督目的，通过察看关键操作、记录测量和运行的数据并核实这些信息，借以持续地掌握材料的库存清单和流向情况的视察机制。(源自：参考文献[4]，11.12)
control center for physical protection	实体保护控制中心【shítǐ bǎohù kòngzhì zhōngxīn】

control sample	对照样品【dùizhào yàngpǐn】
convention	公约【gōngyuē】
Convention on Physical Protection for Nuclear Material The convention signed to promote the peaceful purpose of developing and using nuclear energy among every Nuclear Nonproliferation Treaty State Party, to strengthen the protection of nuclear material usage, storage and transportation, and to prevent the possible dangers caused by illegally obtaining and using nuclear material. It was signed on 3 March, 1980. In July 2005, the amended version of the convention that aims to further strengthen the protection of nuclear material and facilities was adopted and the new convention was signed. The new convention accepted the amendment submitted by China which declared its support for the effort of the international community to strengthen the protection of nuclear facilities, and opposed any form of force or threat of force to any States' peaceful nuclear facility. It also prescribes for the first time that any State Party should further strengthen international cooperation on protecting the safety of nuclear material and preventing nuclear terrorism. (From: Reference[52])	核材料实体(物)保护公约 【hécáiliào shítǐwù bǎohù gōngyuē】 该公约以促进《不扩散核武器条约》的各缔约国和平发展和利用核能为目的，并加强各国对核材料使用、储存和运输的保护，防止核材料的非法获取及使用而可能造成的危险。公约于 1980 年 3 月签署。2005 年 7 月通过了旨在进一步加强核设施与核材料保护的公约修订案并签署了新公约。新公约采纳了中国提交的支持国际社会加强对核设施保护的努力、反对以任何形式对其他国家和平核设施动用武力或进行武力威胁的修订案。新公约还首次明确规定，缔约国要在保护核材料安全、防范核恐怖主义方面进一步加强国际合作。(源自：参考文献[52])
conversion inspection	转化视察【zhuǎnhuà shìchá】
conversion of uranium hexafluoride	六氟化铀转化 【liùfúhuàyóu zhuǎnhuà】
conversion of uranium product	铀产品的转化 【yóuchǎnpǐn de zhuǎnhuà】

E
I
C

conversion plant	转化厂【zhuǎnhuàchǎng】
conversion time The time required to convert different forms of nuclear material to the metallic components of a nuclear explosive device. (From: Reference [4], 3.13)	转化时间【zhuǎnhuà shíjiān】 将不同形式的核材料转化成核爆炸装置金属部件所需要的时间。(源自：参考文献[4]，3.13)
conversion time of nuclear material	核材料转化时间 【hécáiliào zhuǎnhuà shíjiān】
cooling of spent fuel	乏燃料的冷却 【fáránliào de lěngquè】
cooperation protocol	合作议定书【hézuò yìdìngshū】
cooperative security A new security approach that evolved after the end of the Cold War, "which emphasizes reassurance rather than deterrence; it is inclusive rather than exclusive; favours multilateralism over unilateralism or bilateralism; does not rank military solutions over non-military ones; assumes that states are the principal actors in the security system but accepts that non-state actors have an important role to play; does not particularly emphasize the creation of formal security institutions, but does not reject them either; and which, above all, stresses the value of creating habits of dialogue." (From: Reference [65])	合作安全【hézuò ānquán】 冷战后形成的一种新的安全途径，"它强调安全保证，而不是威慑；它是包容性的，而不是排斥性的；它注重多边主义而不是单边或双边主义；它不认为军事手段高于非军事手段；它认为国家是安全体系里的主要行为体，但也接受非国家行为体能发挥重要作用；它不特别强调，但也不拒绝建立正式的安全机构；最重要的是，它强调建立对话习惯的重要性。"(源自：参考文献[65])
Cooperative Threat Reduction Program/Nunn-Lugar Program The November 1991 legislation that provides the Department of Defense (DOD) with the authority to fund assistance to the eligible states of the former Soviet Union to dismantle and	合作减少威胁计划/纳恩-卢格计划 【hézuò jiǎnshǎo wēixié jìhuà nà'ēn lúgé jìhuà】 由美国国会于 1991 年 11 月通过。该立法授权国防部为符合条件的前苏联国家拆除和销毁大规模杀伤性

destroy weapons of mass destruction; to strengthen the security of nuclear weapons and fissile materials in connection with dismantlement; to prevent proliferation; and to help demilitarize the industrial and scientific infrastructure in the Newly Independent States (NIS) which has supported weapons of mass destruction. Since 1996, the Department of State and Department of Energy have assumed responsibility respectively for redirection of weapons expertise and export controls (State) and nuclear material control and accountability (DOE) prog-ram activities. (Modified from: Reference [50])	武器提供资金援助，加强拆卸过程中核武器和裂变材料的安全，防止扩散，帮助独联体国家(NIS)把大规模杀伤性武器的工业和科技基础设施转化为非军事目的。从 1996 年起，美国国务院负责武器专家的转行和出口控制，能源部负责核材料的控制和衡算。(改自：参考文献[50])
core of atomic bomb Refer to "**pit**"	**原子弹弹芯【yuánzǐdàn dànxīn】** 参见"**弹芯**"
CORRTEX (continuous reflectometry for radius vs time experiment)	**科尔太克斯法【kē'ěrtàikèsī fǎ】** (连续反射法测量半径随时间变化的实验)
countercurrent gas centrifuge	**逆流离心机【nìliú líxīnjī】**
counterforce strike The employment of strategic air and missile forces in an effort to destroy, or render impotent, selected military capa-bilities of an enemy force under any of the circumstances by which hostilities may be initiated. (From: Reference [9], p128)	**打击军事力量【dǎjī jūnshì lìliàng】** 在任何可引发冲突的情况下，使用战略空军和导弹力量摧毁或使选定的敌方军事力量失效。(源自：参考文献[9]，p128)
countervalue strike Striking non-military assets of value to the enemy, such as population and industry centers. (Modified from: Reference [27])	**打击社会财富【dǎjī shèhuì cáifù】** 打击敌方有价值的非军事目标，如人口和工业设施。(改自：参考文献[27])

covenant	盟约【méngyuē】
coverage of IAEA safeguards	国际原子能机构保障监督的范围【guójì yuánzǐnéng jīgòu bǎozhàng jiāndū de fànwéi】
cratering of nuclear explosion	核爆炸成坑效应【hébàozhà chéngkēng xiàoyìng】
crisis control A series of interactive processes carried out following the principle of safeguarding national interests and avoiding armed conflicts, to eliminate the factors that may impel the eruption of latent crisis; to lessen the seriousness of the crisis as soon as possible, and to reduce the degree of rivalry and contain the expansion of the crisis. (Modified from: Reference [1], p42)	危机控制【wēijī kòngzhì】 泛指遵循维护国家利益和避免武力冲突的原则而抑制危机扩展的一系列互动过程：在危机尚处潜在阶段时努力消除可能促其爆发的因素；在危机爆发时促其尽快向缓解方向转化，因势利导，尽可能降低对抗程度。(改自：参考文献[1]，p42)
crisis management Procedures for controlling and managing a crisis so that it does not get out of hand and lead to war. Crisis management also ensures that the crisis is resolved so that the vital interests of the states involved are secured and protected. (Modified from: Reference [28], p240)	危机管理【wēijī guǎnlǐ】 控制和管理危机，使其不至于失控而导致战争的过程。危机管理应确保解决危机以保障国家攸关利益。(改自：参考文献[28]，p240)
crisis stability	危机稳定性【wēijī wěndìngxìng】
critical assembly	临界装置【línjiè zhuāngzhì】
criticality safety assessment Analyses and experiments made to ensure fissionable materials used for nuclear weapons remains in a subcritical and safe state during the whole process of production, processing, transportation and assembly. (Modified from: Reference [2], p40)	临界安全评估【línjiè ānquán pínggū】 为确保核武器用的可裂变材料在生产、加工、运输及装配过程中均处于次临界安全状态所进行的实验和分析。(改自：参考文献[2]，p40)

cruise missile	巡航导弹【xúnháng dǎodàn】
cumulative radiation dose	累积辐照剂量【lěijī fúzhào jìliàng】
damaging and injuring effects of shallow or underwater nuclear explosion	水面及水下核爆炸毁伤效应【shuǐmiàn jí shuǐxià hébàozhà huǐshāng xiàoyìng】
damaging and injuring effects of shock wave	冲击波毁伤效应【chōngjībō huǐshāng xiàoyìng】
damaging and injuring effects of surface or underground nuclear explosion	地面或地下核爆炸毁伤效应【dìmiàn huò dìxià hébàozhà huǐshāng xiàoyìng】
damaging and injuring effects of thermal radiation of nuclear explosion	核爆炸光辐射毁伤效应【hébàozhà guāngfúshè huǐshāng xiàoyìng】
data update inspection	数据更新视察【shùjù gēngxīn shìchá】
decay	衰变【shuāibiàn】
decay energy	衰变能【shuāibiànnéng】
declaration	宣言【xuānyán】
decommissioned facility/decommissioned location outside facilities	退役设施/退役的设施外场所【tuìyì shèshī tuìyì de shèshīwài chǎngsuǒ】
decoupled underground nuclear explosion	解耦的地下核爆炸【jiě'ǒu de dìxià hébàozhà】
de-exemption	解除豁免【jiěchú huòmiǎn 】
defect	亏量【kuīliàng】
defense white paper	国防白皮书【guófáng báipíshū】
defensive strategy To guard against and resist the enemy's attack by means of a strategy based on operations that absorb, progressively weaken and block such an attack. (Modified from: Reference [18], p36-37)	防御性战略【fángyùxìng zhànlüè】 在全局上采取承受、逐步削弱和阻止的态势，防备和抗击敌人的进攻。(改自：参考文献[18]，p36-37)
depleted uranium	贫化铀【pínhuàyóu】
depletion	贫化【pínhuà】

design information verification (DIV)	设计资料核查【shèjì zīliào héchá】
destruction	销毁【xiāohuǐ】
destructive analysis (DA)	破坏性分析【pòhuàixìng fēnxī】
detection of nuclear explosion	核爆炸探测【hébàozhà tàncè】
detection probability	探知概率【tànzhī gàilǜ】
detection system for physical protection	实体保护探测系统【shítǐ bǎohù tàncè xìtǒng】
detection system of nuclear explosion	核爆炸探测系统【hébàozhà tàncè xìtǒng】
detection technology of nuclear explosion	核爆炸探测技术【hébàozhà tàncè jìshù】
detection time	探知时间【tànzhī shíjiān】
detente	缓和【huǎnhé】
deterrence The prevention from action by fear of the consequences. Deterrence is a state of mind brought about by the existence of a credible threat of unacceptable counteraction. (From: Reference [9], p160) Refer to "**compellence**"	威慑【wēishè】 通过使对手害怕后果来防止其采取行动。威慑是一种由难以承受的反击行动所致的可信威胁的存在所引发的心理状态。(源自：参考文献[9]，p160) 参见"**威逼**"
deterrence of diversion	遏制转用【èzhì zhuǎnyòng】
deuterium	氘【dāo】
diagnostic and measurement of nuclear test	核试验的诊断和测量【héshìyàn de zhěnduàn hé cèliáng】
diffuser	扩散分离器【kuòsàn fēnlíqì】
diffusion barrier	分离膜【fēnlímó】
diffusion separation unit	扩散分离机组【kuòsàn fēnlí jīzǔ】
directed-energy weapon driven by a nuclear explosion	核爆激励定向能武器【hébào jīlì dìngxiàngnéng wǔqì】

direct-use material Nuclear material that can be used for the manufacture of nuclear explosive devices without transmutation or further enrichment. (From: Reference [4], 4.25)	**直接使用材料【zhíjiē shǐyòng cáiliào】** 未经嬗变或进一步浓缩就可用于制造核爆炸装置的核材料。(源自：参考文献[4]，4.25)
dirty bomb Refer to "**radiological dispersal device (RDD)**"	**脏弹【zāngdàn】** 参见"**放射性物质散布装置**"
disarmament	**裁军【cáijūn】**
dissuasion In current U.S. thinking, "to persuade other powers to refrain from initiating a competition in military capabilities." (From: Reference [41]) Note: In the context of nuclear doctrine, the French word, "la dissuasion" means essentially "deterrence". (From: Reference [69], pII-41)	**劝阻【quànzǔ】** 在当前美国思维中，指劝说其他大国放弃与美国在军事能力方面的竞争。(源自：参考文献[41]) 注：在核学说范畴，法语单词"la dissuasion"实质上意指威慑。(源自：参考文献[69]，pII-41)
distinguishability exhibition	**可区分性展示【kěqūfēnxìng zhǎnshì】**
diversion of nuclear material	**核材料转用【hécáiliào zhuǎnyòng】**
diversion strategy/diversion path A (hypothetical) scheme which a State could consider to divert nuclear material or to misuse items subject to IAEA safeguards. Diversion strategies would include: the undeclared removal of nuclear material from a safeguarded facility or the use of a safeguarded facility for the introduction, production or processing of undeclared nuclear material. (From: Reference [4], 3.7)	**转用策略/转用途径【zhuǎnyòng cèlüè zhuǎnyòng tújìng】** 一种(假定的)策略，即某国可能考虑转用国际原子能机构保障监督的核材料或不正当使用国际原子能机构保障监督的物项。转用策略可能包括：从一个受保障监督的设施内擅自转移核材料或利用一个受保障监督的核设施引进、生产或处理未申报的核材料。(源自：参考文献[4]，3.7)

diversity of technical protection systems	技术防护系统的多样性【jìshù fánghù xìtǒng de duōyàngxìng】
doctrine of "reasonable sufficiency"	“合理足够”原则【hélǐ zúgòu yuánzé】
downstream facility	下游设施【xiàyóu shèshī】
drilling to obtain radioactive samples	钻探取样【zuāntàn qǔyàng】
dry reprocessing	干法后处理【gānfǎ hòuchǔlǐ】
dry storage	干法贮存【gānfǎ zhùcún】
DUPIC (Direct Use of Spent PWR fuel in CANDU reactors) process	杜皮克工艺【dùpíkè gōngyì】(压水堆乏燃料直接用于坎杜反应堆的工艺)
early-warning satellite	预警卫星【yùjǐng wèixīng】
effects of nuclear explosion on communication	核爆炸通信效应【hébàozhà tōngxìn xiàoyìng】
effects of radioactive contamination	放射性沾染效应【fàngshèxìng zhānrǎn xiàoyìng】
efficiency of barrier The ratio of a porous barrier's real enrichment factor to its theoretical maximum enrichment factor. Because of non-ideal molecular flow and back diffusion, the real enrichment factor is less than the theoretical maximum enrichment factor. (Modified from: Reference [2], p126)	分离膜效率【fēnlímó xiàolǜ】 分离膜的实际浓缩因子与理想浓缩因子的比值。由于非纯分子流和膜后反扩散的影响，分离膜的实际浓缩因子通常小于理想浓缩因子。(改自：参考文献[2]，p126)
efficiency of cascade	级联效率【jílián xiàolǜ】
Eighteen-Nation Committee on Disarmament (ENCD)	十八国裁军委员会【shíbāguó cáijūn wěiyuánhuì】
electromagnetic-pulse boundary-wave type simulator	有界波型电磁脉冲模拟器【yǒujiè bōxíng diàncí màichōng mónǐqì】
electromagnetic pulse of high-altitude nuclear explosion	高空核爆炸电磁脉冲【gāokōng hébàozhà diàncí màichōng】

electromagnetic-pulse radiation-wave type simulator	辐射波型电磁脉冲模拟器【fúshèbōxíng diàncí màichōng móňǐqì】
electromagnetic pulse weapon A nuclear explosive designed to enhance the electromagnetic pulse radiated by a nuclear weapon. (From: Reference [20])	电磁脉冲弹【diàncí màichōng dàn】一种设计成能加强核武器电磁脉冲效应的核爆炸装置。(源自：参考文献[20])
electromagnetic pulse weapon driven by nuclear explosion	核爆驱动电磁脉冲弹【hébào qūdòng diàncí màichōngdàn】
electron	电子【diànzǐ】
electron gun	电子枪【diànzǐqiāng】
electronic reconnaissance satellite/electronic intelligence (ELINT) satellite	电子侦察卫星【diànzǐ zhēnchá wèixīng】
elimination inspection	销毁视察【xiāohuǐ shìchá】
ending inventory of nuclear material	核材料末期存量【hécáiliào mòqī cúnliàng】
energy consumption of unit separative work	单位分离功能耗【dānwèi fēnlígōng nénghào】
engineering design of nuclear weapon	核武器工程设计【héwǔqì gōngchéng shèjì】
enhanced X-ray weapon	增强 **X** 射线弹【zēngqiáng **X** shèxiàndàn】
enriched uranium	浓缩(富集)铀【nóngsuō fùjí yóu】
enrichment	浓缩(富集)度【nóngsuō fùjí dù】
enrichment factor	浓缩(富集)因子【nóngsuō fùjí yīnzǐ】
enrichment plant/isotope separation plant	浓缩(富集)厂/同位素分离厂【nóngsuō fùjí chǎng tóngwèisù fēnlíchǎng】
entrance and exit control	出入口控制【chūrùkǒu kòngzhì】

E I C

environmental sampling In the context of IAEA safeguards, the collection of samples from the environment with a view to analyzing them for traces of materials that can reveal information about nuclear material handled or activities conducted. (From: Reference [4], 9.1)	环境取样【huánjìng qǔyàng】 在 IAEA 保障监督框架内，从环境中取样，并通过对样品的分析获取相关痕迹以揭示所处理的核材料或进行的活动的信息。(源自：参考文献[4]，9.1)
environmental sampling of nuclear explosion	核爆炸环境取样 【hébàozhà huánjìng qǔyàng】
environmental simulation test of nuclear weapon	核武器环境模拟试验 【héwǔqì huánjìng mónǐ shìyàn】
equipment for ground test and monitoring of nuclear weapon	核武器地面测控设备 【héwǔqì dìmiàn cèkòng shèbèi】
equivalent dose	当量剂量【dāngliàng jìliàng】
equivalent megatonnage The 2/3 power of the yield of a nuclear warhead measured by megaton TNT equivalent. The formula is $EMT=(Y/Y_0)^{2/3}$, where Y is the yield of a nuclear warhead and Y_0 is one megaton TNT equivalent. (Modified from: Reference [3], p115-116)	等效百万吨数 【děngxiào báiwàndūnshù】 以百万吨 TNT 当量为单位计量核弹威力的数值的三分之二次方。用公式可表示为 $EMT=(Y/Y_0)^{2/3}$。式中 Y 为核弹威力，Y_0 为一百万吨 TNT 当量。(改自：参考文献[3]，p115-116)
equivalent megatonnage-to-weight ratio	比等效百万吨数 【bǐděngxiào bǎiwàndūnshù】
error	误差【wùchā】
essential equipment list (EEL)	重要设备清单 【zhòngyào shèbèi qīngdān】
examine and repair deployed warhead	部署弹头的检修 【bùshǔ dàntóu de jiǎnxiū】
exchange of notes	换文【huànwén】
exemption from IAEA safeguards	国际原子能机构保障监督的豁免 【guójì yuánzǐnéng jīgòu bǎozhàng jiāndū de huòmiǎn】

existing stock of nuclear material	核材料现有库存【hécáiliào xiànyǒu kùcún】
exposure	照射【zhàoshè】
extended nuclear deterrence 1 Strategy of preventing nuclear attack on one's allies by threatening the perceived or potential enemy with unacceptable damage by nuclear retaliation. 2 Strategy of preventing conventional attack on oneself or one's allies by threat of nuclear retaliation. (Modified from: Reference [7], p14-15)	延伸(扩展)核威慑【yánshēn kuòzhǎn héwēishè】 1 通过用核报复导致无法承受的毁伤以威胁觉察到的或潜在的敌手，防止其对盟国进行核打击的战略。 2 以威胁核报复来防止对其或其盟友进行常规打击的战略。(改自：参考文献[7]，p14-15)
false-alarm rate The ratio of alarms triggered by real events to the total number of alarms the monitoring system detects. The false alarms are generated because the monitoring system could not distinguish real from false alarms. (Modified from: Reference [1], p489)	虚警率【xūjǐnglǜ】 被非真实事件驱动的报警次数与监测系统设计上所能侦测到的总报警次数的比例。虚警的产生是由于监测系统无法区分真实的或虚假的警报。(改自：参考文献[1]，p489)
fast-neutron criticality facility	快中子临界装置【kuàizhōngzǐ línjiè zhuāngzhì】
fast-neutron pulse reactor	快中子脉冲堆【kuàizhōngzǐ màichōng duī】
fast neutrons	快中子【kuàizhōngzǐ】
fast reactor	快堆【kuàiduī】
feed and withdrawals of a gas centrifuge	气体离心机的供取料【qìtǐ líxīnjī de gōngqǔliào】
feed material	供料【gōngliào】
fertile material Nuclear material that can be converted into a special fissionable material through capture of one neutron per nucleus. (From: Reference [4], 4.7)	可转换材料【kězhuǎnhuàn cáiliào】 通过在一个原子核中俘获一个中子而能被转化为特种可裂变材料的一种核材料。(源自：参考文献[4]，4.7)

Final Document of the Special Session of the General Assembly Devoted to Disarmament	联大裁军特别会议最后文件【liándà cáijūn tèbié huìyì zuìhòu wénjiàn】
firing range	射程【shèchéng】
firing the nuclear weapon	核武器引爆【héwǔqì yǐnbào】
First Committee of the UN General Assembly	联合国大会第一委员会【liánhéguó dàhuì dìyī wěiyuánhuì】
first-generation nuclear weapon	第一代核武器【dìyīdài héwǔqì】
fissile material	易裂变材料【yìlièbiàn cáiliào】
fission neutrons	裂变中子【lièbiàn zhōngzǐ】
fission weapon	裂变武器【lièbiàn wǔqì】
fission yield	裂变产额/裂变威力【lièbiàn chǎn'é lièbiàn wēilì】
fissionable material In general, an isotope or a mixture of isotopes capable of nuclear fission. Some fissionable materials are capable of fission only by sufficiently fast neutrons (e.g. neutrons of a kinetic energy above 1 MeV). Isotopes that undergo fission by neutrons of all energies, including slow (thermal) neutrons, are usually referred to as fissile materials or fissile isotopes. For example, isotopes U-233, U-235, Pu-239 and Pu-241 are referred to as both fissionable and fissile, while U-236 and Pu-240 are fissionable but not fissile. (From: Reference[4], 4.6)	可裂变材料【kělièbiàn cáiliào】 一般而言，指能产生核裂变的一种同位素或同位素混合物。有些可裂变材料只有在足够快的中子(如动能超过 1 MeV 的中子)作用下才能发生裂变。在所有能量的中子包括慢(热)中子作用下都可以发生裂变的同位素通常称之为易裂变材料或易裂变同位素。例如，同位素 铀-233，铀-235，钚-239，钚-241 既被称为可裂变材料又被称为易裂变材料，而铀-238 和钚-240 仅被称为可裂变材料而不是易裂变材料。(源自：参考文献[4]，4.6)
Five Principles of Peaceful Coexistence The Five Principles are: mutual respect	和平共处五项原则【hépíng gòngchǔ wǔxiàng yuánzé】 和平共处五项原则，即相互尊重主

E
C

for sovereignty and territorial integrity, mutual non-aggression, non-interference in each other's internal affairs, equality and mutual benefit, and peaceful coexistence. In negotiation with an Indian delegation the Five Principles were set forth by Premier Zhou Enlai, and subsequently included in the joint communique issued by Premier Zhou Enlai and Prime Minister Jawaharlal Nehru, in June 1954. Since that time the principles have been adopted in many other international documents. (Modified from: Reference[53])	权和领土完整、互不侵犯、互不干涉内政、平等互利、和平共处。这五项原则由周恩来总理在与印度代表团谈判时提出，并于 1954 年 6 月首次被写入周恩来总理与贾瓦哈·尼赫鲁总理签署的联合公报中，此后被众多国际性文件所采用并成为公认的指导国际关系的准则。(源自：参考文献[53])
flash radiography by pulsed X-ray system	闪光 X 射线照相【shǎnguāng X shèxiàn zhàoxiàng】
flow field in gas centrifuge	气体离心机流场【qìtǐ líxīnjī liúchǎng】
fluoride volatility process	氟化挥发法【fúhuà huīfāfǎ】
fluorides of uranium	铀的氟化物【yóu de fúhuàwù】
fluorination of uranium oxide	铀氧化物的氟化【yóuyǎnghuàwù de fúhuà】
focusing of weak shock wave	弱冲击波聚焦【ruò chōngjībō jùjiāo】
formerly declared facility inspection	先前申报设施视察【xiānqián shēnbào shèshī shìchá】
forward defense strategy	前沿防御战略【qiányán fángyù zhànlüè】
fratricidal effect of nuclear weapon	核武器自相摧毁效应【héwǔqì zìxiāng cuīhuǐ xiàoyìng】
freeze	冻结【dòngjié】
fuel assembly	燃料组件【ránliào zǔjiàn】
fuel bundle	燃料棒束【ránliàobàngshù】
fuel component	燃料部件【ránliào bùjiàn】

fuel element	燃料元件【ránliào yuánjiàn】
fuel fabrication plant	燃料制造厂【ránliào zhìzàochǎng】
fuel of fusion	聚变燃料【jùbiàn ránliào】
fusion reaction	聚变反应【jùbiàn fǎnyìng】
fusion yield	聚变威力【jùbiàn wēilì】
fuze of nuclear weapon	核武器引信【héwǔqì yǐnxìn】
G-8 Global Partnership Against the Spread of Weapons and Materials of Mass Destruction Launched in 2002 by the G-8 (Russian, the U.S., Britian, France, Japan, Germany, Canada and Italy), this effort aims to prevent the proliferation of weapons of mass destruction to terrorists or those who support them through projects pertaining to disarmament, nonproliferation, counterterrorism and nuclear safety. Originally targeted at carrying out $20 billion of projects in Russia over 10 years, the G-8 Global Partnership has expanded to include additional countries. (Modified from: References [42-43])	八国集团“防止大规模杀伤性武器和材料扩散的全球伙伴计划”【bāguó jítuán fángzhǐ dàguīmó shāshāngxìng wǔqì hé cáiliào kuòsàn de quánqiú huǒbàn jìhuà】 该计划是八国集团(俄罗斯、美国、英国、法国、日本、德国、加拿大和意大利)于 2002 年提出的，旨在通过与裁军、不扩散、反恐和核安全有关的项目，防止大规模杀伤性武器扩散到恐怖主义者或其支持者手中。最初目标是在俄罗斯开展为期 10 年耗资 200 亿美元的项目，现八国集团全球伙伴关系已经扩展到八国以外的国家。(改自：参考文献 [42-43])
gamma radiation monitoring and energy spectrum analysis	γ辐射监测和能谱分析【γ fúshè jiāncè hé néngpǔ fēnxī】
gas centrifuge	气体离心机【qìtǐ líxīnjī】
gaseous diffusion method	气体扩散法【qìtǐ kuòsànfǎ】
gaseous diffusion plant	气体扩散工厂【qìtǐ kuòsàn gōngchǎng】
geological repository	地质处置库【dìzhì chǔzhìkù】
geophysical effects of nuclear explosion	核爆炸地球物理效应【hébàozhà dìqiúwùlǐ xiàoyìng】

geophysical survey in on-site inspections	现场视察中的地球物理勘测【xiànchǎng shìchá zhōng de dìqiú wùlǐ kāncè】
glass solidification	玻璃固化【bōli gùhuà】
Global Initiative to Combat Nuclear Terrorism Launched in 2006 by the United States and Russia, the initiative aims to prevent terrorist access to nuclear materials by improving accounting and security of radioactive and nuclear materials, enhancing security at civilian nuclear facilities, and improving detection of nuclear and radioactive materials to prevent illicit trafficking. (From: Reference [44])	打击核恐怖主义全球行动倡议【dǎjī hékǒngbùzhǔyì quánqiú xíngdòng chàngyì】 2006年由美国和俄国发起，旨在防止恐怖主义分子获取核材料的倡议，具体措施包括：改善核及放射性材料的衡算与安全，加强对民用核设施的保护，提高对核及放射性物质探测能力以防止非法走私。(源自：参考文献[44])
global strategy Strategy that aims at achieving and maintaining global interests for a nation or a group of nations through military, economic, political, diplomatic and other means. (From: Reference [1], p25)	全球战略【quánqiú zhànlüè】 泛指运用军事、经济、政治、外交等手段以实现和保护国家或国家集团在全球的利益的方略。(源自：参考文献[1]，p25)
glove box	手套箱【shǒutàoxiāng】
graphite moderated reactor	石墨慢化堆【shímò mànhuàduī】
gravimetric analysis	重量分析【zhòngliàng fēnxī】
green salt The popular name of green uranium tetrafluoride (UF_4) crystal. It is an important mid-point production in the process of producing uranium fuel. It can be used to produce uranium hexafluoride (UF_6) and uranium metal. (From: Reference [2], p304)	绿盐【lǜyán】 绿色的 UF_4 晶体，是铀工艺中 UF_4 的俗称。UF_4 是生产核燃料的重要中间产品，用于制备六氟化铀(UF_6)和金属铀。(源自：参考文献[2]，p304)
ground resolution/spatial resolution	地面分辨率/空间分辨率【dìmiàn fēnbiànlǜ kōngjiān fēnbiànlǜ】

ground zero	爆心投影点【bàoxīn tóuyǐngdiǎn】
Group of 21	21 国集团【èrshíyīguó jítuán】
Guidelines for the Management of Plutonium The Guidelines adopted by nine states (the five nuclear weapon states and Germany, Japan, Belgium and Switzerland) in 1997, with a view to ensuring that holdings of plutonium are managed safely and effectively in accordance with international commitments, including their obligations under the NPT (and, for states that are members of the European Community, also under the Euratom Treaty), and with their safeguards agreements with the IAEA. The Guidelines describe, inter alia, the nuclear material accountancy system, physical protection measures and international transfer procedures applicable to the plutonium subject to the Guidelines. They further specify the information to be published by the participating States in respect of plutonium management, including annual statements of their holdings of civil unirradiated plutonium and of their estimates of plutonium contained in spent civil reactor fuel. (From: Reference [1], p409; [4], 1.30)	钚管理指导原则 【bù guǎnlǐ zhǐdǎo yuánzé】 该指导原则由五个核武器国家和德国、日本、比利时、瑞士等九国于 1997 年通过，它着眼于按照国际约定(包括它们在 NPT 下的义务，欧共体成员国还有欧洲原子能联营条约下的义务)和 IAEA 的保障监督协定确保对持有的钚进行安全有效的管理。该指导原则描述了在接受该指导原则下适用于钚的核材料衡算体制、实体保护措施和国际运输手续。它还进一步指定了参与国要发布的有关钚管理的信息，包括他们所持有的民用未辐照钚和民用反应堆乏燃料中含有的钚估量的年度申报。(源自：参考文献[1]，p409；[4]，1.30)
gun-type atomic bomb	枪法原子弹【qiāngfǎ yuánzǐdàn】
half-life	半衰期【bànshuāiqī】
hardened target	加固目标【jiāgù mùbiāo】
heavy water	重水【zhòngshuǐ】

heavy water production plant	重水生产厂 【zhòngshuǐ shēngchǎnchǎng】
heavy water reactor (HWR)	重水堆【zhòngshuǐduī】
hedge warheads stockpile One part of the U.S. active stockpile of warheads, retained as part of the responsive force, to be used to augment the operationally deployed force in order to meet potential contingencies, unanticipated events or emerging threats. (Modified from: Reference [66], p4; [67-68])	备用性核武库【bèiyòngxìng héwǔkù】 美国现役核武库的一部分，作为响应力量的一部分予以保留，用来加强作战部署的力量以应对潜在的意外事故、突发的事件或显现的威胁。(改自：参考文献[66] p4，[67-68])
hedging strategy A balanced approach to foster cooperation with a nation where possible while also preparing for hostile activity. (Modified from: Reference [45])	两面下注战略 【liǎngmiàn xiàzhù zhànlüè】 尽可能促进和他国合作但也为敌对活动做准备的一种均衡做法。(改自：参考文献[45])
hegemonism	霸权主义【bàquánzhǔyì】
helium-3	氦-3【hài sān】
high-enriched uranium (HEU)	高浓铀【gāonóngyóu】
high level radioactive waste	高放废物【gāofàngfèiwù】
high resolution sensing camera	高分辨率灵敏照相机 【gāofēnbiànlǜ língmǐn zhàoxiàngjī】
high-technology warfare	高技术战争【gāojìshù zhànzhēng】
high temperature gas-cooled reactor (HTGR)	高温气冷堆【gāowēn qìlěngduī】
hold-up	滞留量【zhìliúliàng】
hot cell	热室【rèshì】
hydroacoustic monitoring	水声监测【shuǐshēng jiāncè】
hydrodynamic experiment An experiment used to simulate the implosion process of a nuclear explosive. It uses other materials such	流体动力学实验 【liútǐ dònglìxué shíyàn】 为模拟核爆炸内爆过程所进行的实验。它是用代用材料(如铀-238、钨、

as U-238, tungsten and steel as substitute for fissile materials such as HEU or Pu-239 in a nuclear device, and uses the high explosive to compress the whole or partial structure of the device. As the materials are in the liquid state under the compression of explosion of high explosive, such experiments are called hydrodynamic experiments. The experiment releases no nuclear energy and is not required to be conducted at a nuclear test site. (From: Reference [1], p212-213)	钢等)替代核装置中的裂变材料高浓铀或钚-239、用高能炸药爆炸压缩该装置的整体或部分结构而进行的一种实验。由于装置中的材料在高能炸药爆炸压缩下处于流体状态，因此称此类实验为流体动力学实验。这种实验没有核能释放，实验不一定要在核试验场地进行。(源自：参考文献[1]，p212-213)
hydrogen bomb	氢弹【qīngdàn】
hydronuclear experiment A method for assessing some aspects of nuclear weapon safety, first conducted at Los Alamos during the 1958-61 moratorium on nuclear testing to investigate the "one-point" safety of a nuclear explosive. The experiments resulted in subcritical multiplying assemblies or a very slight degree of supercriticality and, in some cases, involved a fission energy release less than the design limit of 7 megajoules. (Modified from: Reference [30], p1)	流体核实验【liútǐ héshíyàn】 一种评估核武器某些安全问题的方法，由洛斯·阿拉莫斯国家实验室(LANL)在 1958 年至 1961 年的暂停核试验期间研究核爆炸"一点安全"时首先使用。该实验在次临界增殖装置中或极轻微的超临界状态下进行，在某些情况下会释放小于 7 兆焦设计限额的裂变能。(改自：参考文献[30]，p1)
IAEA inspection goal	国际原子能机构视察指标 【guójì yuánzǐnéng jīgòu shìchá zhǐbiāo】
IAEA Safeguards System	国际原子能机构的保障监督体系 【guójì yuánzǐnéng jīgòu de bǎozhàng jiāndū tǐxì】
IAEA timeliness detection goal	国际原子能机构及时性探知指标 【guójì yuánzǐnéng jīgòu jíshíxìng tànzhī zhǐbiāo】
IAEA's 93+2 program	国际原子能机构"93+2"计划 【guójì yuánzǐnéng jīgòu "93+2" jìhuà】

E I C

ideal separation factor of gaseous diffusion process	气体扩散的理想分离因子 【qìtǐ kuòsàn de lǐxiǎng fēnlí yīnzǐ】
identity (identification) data	标识数据【biāoshí shùjù】
imaging reconnaissance satellite	成像侦察卫星 【chéngxiàng zhēnchá wèixīng】
implosion-type atomic bomb	内爆法原子弹 【nèibàofǎ yuánzǐdàn】
inactive nuclear stockpile	非现役核武库【fēi xiànyì héwǔkù】
inactive warhead	非现役弹头【fēi xiànyì dàntóu】
indirect use material All nuclear material except direct use material. It includes: depleted, natural and low enriched uranium, and thorium, all of which must be further processed in order to produce direct use material. (From: Reference [4], 4.26)	非直接使用材料 【fēi zhíjiē shǐyòng cáiliào】 除直接使用材料以外的所有核材料。它包括：贫化铀、天然铀和低浓缩铀以及钍，所有这些材料都必须经过进一步加工以生产直接使用材料。(源自：参考文献[4]，4.26)
induced-radioactivity bomb A type of hydrogen bomb that utilizes radioisotopes induced by neutrons during a nuclear explosion to increase radioactive contamination. In February 1950 Hungarian physicist Leo Szilard published the concept of this bomb — the "cobalt bomb". However no state manufactures and tests this kind of bomb. (From: Reference [2], p63)	感生放射性弹 【gǎnshēng fàngshèxìngdàn】 利用核爆中子感生的放射性同位素增大放射性沾染的一种氢弹。1950 年 2 月匈牙利物理学家 L・西拉德最早提出这种弹的设想——“钴弹”。但并没有人制造和试验。(源自：参考文献[2]，p63)
inertia fuze of nuclear weapon	核武器惯性引信 【héwǔqì guànxìng yǐnxìn】
inertial confinement fusion (ICF)	惯性约束聚变 【guànxìng yuēshù jùbiàn】
INFCIRC/153 safeguards agreement (IAEA)	**INFCIRC/153 型保障监督协定 (IAEA)** 【INFCIRC 153 xíng bǎozhàng jiāndū xiédìng】

E
I
C

INFCIRC/66 safeguards agreement (IAEA)	**INFCIRC/66 型保障监督协定 (IAEA)** 【INFCIRC 66 xíng bǎozhàng jiāndū xiédìng】
information barrier Used to protect any sensitive weapon design information that may be gathered during the identification process, for example, by automating the collection, storage, and analysis of data, and by making only the conclusions of the analysis available to the inspector. (Modified from: Reference [11], p107-108)	信息屏障【xìnxī píngzhàng】 用来保护鉴别过程中可能搜集到的敏感武器设计信息。这可以通过自动进行采集、储存和分析数据，并只向视察员提供分析的结果来实现。(改自：参考文献[11]，p107-108)
information warfare (IW)	信息战【xìnxīzhàn】
infrared remote sensor	红外遥感器【hóngwài yáogǎnqì】
infrasound monitoring	次声监测【cìshēng jiāncè】
initial inspection	初始视察【chūshǐ shìchá】
initial nuclear radiation of nuclear explosion	核爆炸早期核辐射 【hébàozhà zǎoqī héfúshè】
initial physical inventory of nuclear material	核材料初始存量 【hécáiliào chūshǐ cúnliàng】
initiating component	起爆元件【qǐbào yuánjiàn】
initiating sequence	起爆序列【qǐbào xùliè】
injuring and damaging effects of initial nuclear radiation of nuclear explosion	核爆炸早期核辐射毁伤效应 【hébàozhà zǎoqī héfúshè huǐshāng xiàoyìng】
insensitive high explosive	钝感高能炸药 【dùngǎn gāonéng zhàyào】
integral process	一体化流程【yītǐhuà liúchéng】
integrated numerical simulation experiment of explosion device	核(爆炸)装置全过程数值模拟实验 【hé bàozhà zhuāngzhì quánguòchéng shùzhí mónǐ shíyàn】
integrated safeguards The optimum combination of all	一体化保障监督 【yītǐhuà bǎozhàng jiāndū】

safeguards measures available to the IAEA under comprehensive safeguards agreements and additional protocols to achieve maximum effectiveness and efficiency in meeting the IAEA's safeguards obligations within available resources. (From: Reference [4], 3.5)	在全面保障监督协议及附加议定书下，国际原子能机构所能获得的所有保障监督手段的最佳组合，其目的是利用可拥有的资源，最有效、最高效地满足国际原子能机构规定的保障监督义务。(源自：参考文献[4]，3.5)
integrated test of Arming, Fuzing & Firing (AF&F) system	引控系统联试【yǐnkòng xìtǒng liánshì】
integrity of protection system	保护系统完整性【bǎohù xìtǒng wánzhěngxìng】
Interim Agreement Between the United States of America and the Union of Soviet Socialist Republics on Certain Measures with Respect to the Limitation of Strategic Offensive Arms (SALT I)	美苏限制进攻性战略武器的某些措施的临时协定【měi sū xiànzhì jìngōngxìng zhànlüè wǔqì de mǒuxiē cuòshī de línshí xiédìng】
intermediate fluorides of uranium	铀的中间氟化物【yóu de zhōngjiān fúhuàwù】
intermediate-level radioactive waste	中放废物【zhōngfàng fèiwù】
intermediate product	中间产品【zhōngjiān chǎnpǐn】
International Atomic Energy Agency (IAEA)	国际原子能机构【guójì yuánzǐnéng jīgòu】
international conflict	国际冲突【guójì chōngtū】
international custom	国际惯例【guójì guànlì】
International Data Center (IDC)	国际数据中心【guójì shùjù zhōngxīn】
international dispute	国际争端【guójì zhēngduān】
international law	国际法【guójìfǎ】
International Maritime Organization (IMO)	国际海事组织【guójì hǎishì zǔzhī】
International Monitoring System (IMS)	国际监测系统【guójì jiāncè xìtǒng】

Part of the verification system that was established to verify the implementation of the Comprehensive Nuclear Test Ban Treaty (CTBT). It mainly consists of a seismic monitoring network, an atmospheric radionuclide monitoring network, an infrasound monitoring network and a hydroacoustic monitoring network. (From: Reference [1], p478)	为核查《全面禁止核试验条约》(CTBT)执行情况而建立的核查机制的一个组成部分。它主要由地震监测网、大气放射性核素监测网、次声监测网和水声监测网组成。(源自：参考文献[1]，p478)
international sanction	国际制裁【guójì zhìcái】
international standards of accountancy	国际衡算标准 【guójì héngsuàn biāozhǔn】
international strategic pattern	国际战略格局【guójì zhànlüè géjú】
international technical means (for verification)	国际技术手段(核查用) 【guójì jìshù shǒuduàn hécháyòng】
international treaty	国际条约【guójì tiáoyuē】
inventory	存量【cúnliàng】
inventory change	存量变化【cúnliàng biànhuà】
ion	离子【lízǐ】
isotope	同位素【tóngwèisù】
isotope separation	同位素分离【tóngwèisù fēnlí】
isotope separation factor A characteristic value for measuring separative efficiency of a separative unit. It is the ratio of the relative concentration after and before processing. (From: Reference [2], p404)	同位素分离因子 【tóngwèisù fēnlí yīnzǐ】 表征分离单元分离效果的特征量，表示某一分离效应所产生同位素相对丰度的变化情况。(源自：参考文献[2]，p404)
isotope shift	同位素位移【tóngwèisù wèiyí】
item counting	物件计数【wùjiàn jìshù】
Joint Statement by the President of the People's	中华人民共和国主席和俄罗斯联邦总统关于互不首先使用核武器和互

Republic of China and the President of the Russian Federation on No-First-Use of Nuclear Weapons and Detargeting of Strategic Nuclear Weapons Against Each Other	不将战略核武器瞄准对方的联合声明 【zhōnghuá rénmín gònghéguó zhǔxí hé éluósī liánbāng zǒngtǒng guānyú hùbù shǒuxiān shǐyòng héwǔqì hé hùbù jiāng zhànlüèhéwǔqì miáozhǔn duìfāng de liánhé shēngmíng】
key measurement point (KMP)	关键测量点【guānjiàn cèliángdiǎn】
kill probability	毁伤概率【huǐshāng gàilǜ】
laser chemical isotope separation	激光化学法分离同位素 【jīguāng huàxuéfǎ fēnlí tóngwèisù】
laser isotope separation	激光分离同位素 【jīguāng fēnlí tóngwèisù】
laser plasma ion extraction	激光等离子体离子萃取 【jīguāng děnglízǐtǐlízǐ cuìqǔ】
launch-on-warning (LOW)	预警即发射【yùjǐng jì fāshè】
launch-under-attack (LUA)	遇袭即发射【yùxí jì fāshè】
lifespan of nuclear weapon The whole period of a nuclear weapon's life, beginning from when it was produced until when it could no longer fulfill technical performance criteria or meet operational requirements. (Modified from: Reference [2], p222)	核武器寿命【héwǔqì shòumìng】 核武器从出厂到无法满足技术性能指标和作战使用要求的整个过程的期限。(改自：参考文献[2]，p222)
lifetime extension and decommissioning of nuclear weapon	核武器的延寿与退役 【héwǔqì de yánshòu yǔ tuìyì】
light water reactor (LWR)	轻水堆【qīngshuǐduī】
limited deterrence A term used by some scholars to describe a form of deterrence. However, there is no consensus on the definition. Note 1: In some descriptions limited deterrence requires a limited warfight-	有限威慑【yǒuxiàn wēishè】 某些学者用于描述某种威慑形式所用的术语，但目前尚无定论。 注 1：在有些描述中，有限威慑要求有一定的核战能力，能够在核战

ing capability to inflict costly damage on the adversary at every rung on the escalation ladder, thus denying the adversary victory in a nuclear war. (Modified from: Reference [46]) Note 2: In some descriptions it refers to France's nuclear deterrent. (Modified from: Reference [18], p360; [70], p195-196) Note 3: "deterrence" can also apply in non-nuclear circumstances.	争中的各升级阶梯上给对手造成损失，从而挫败对手使之不能取胜。(改自：参考文献[46]) 注 2：在有些描述中是指法国的核威慑。(改自：参考文献[18]，p360；[70]，p195-196) 注 3："威慑"亦适应于非核情况。
limited war	有限战争【yǒuxiàn zhànzhēng】
limit	限制【xiànzhì】
lithium	锂【lǐ】
lithium deuteride	氘化锂【dāohuàlǐ】
lithium deutero-tritide	氘氚化锂【dāochuānhuàlǐ】
lithium hydride	氢化锂【qīnghuàlǐ】
lithium isotopes separation	锂同位素分离【lǐ tóngwèisù fēnlí】
local war	局部战争【júbù zhànzhēng】
location outside facilities (LOF)	设施外场所【shèshīwài chǎngsuǒ】
long-term biological effects of nuclear explosion	核爆炸的长期生物效应【hébàozhà de chángqī shēngwù xiàoyìng】
low-enriched uranium (LEU)	低浓铀【dīnóngyóu】
low level radioactive waste	低放废物【dīfàng fèiwù】
maintainability of nuclear weapon	核武器可维修性【héwǔqì kěwéixiūxìng】
managed access Upon the request of a State, the IAEA and the State shall make arrangements for managed access, arranged in such a way as "to prevent the dissemination of proliferation sensitive information, to meet safety or physical protection	限制准入【xiànzhì zhǔnrù】 指在被视察国的要求下，IAEA 和该国达成的限制进入权限的安排。这种安排应按照"防止与扩散相关的敏感信息的散布、满足安全或实体保护要求或者保护所有权或商业

requirements, or to protect proprietary or commercially sensitive information." (From: Reference [4], 11.26)	敏感信息"的原则制定。(源自：参考文献[4]，11.26)
maneuverable reentry vehicle (MaRV)	机动再入弹头【jīdòng zàirù dàntóu】
marine propulsion reactor	舰船用动力反应堆【jiànchuányòng dònglì fǎnyìngduī】
material balance area (MBA)	核材料平衡区【hécáiliào pínghéngqū】
material balance period (MBP)	材料平衡周期【cáiliào pínghéng zhōuqī】
material category	材料类别【cáiliào lèibié】
material description	材料说明【cáiliào shuōmíng】
material form	材料形态【cáiliào xíngtài】
material type	材料类型【cáiliào lèixíng】
material unaccounted for (MUF)	不明材料量【bùmíng cáiliàoliàng】
maximum deterrence A term used in the past by some Chinese military scholars to describe a form of deterrence whereby with strong nuclear superiority as support, the threat of a massive nuclear strike is used to deter the adversary. (Modified from: Reference [18], p359) Refer to "**deterrence**"	最大核威慑【zuìdà héwēishè】 部分中国军事学者以前描述一种核威慑形式所使用的术语，即用强大的核优势为后盾，以大规模使用核武器作威胁来威慑对手。(改自：参考文献[18]，p359) 参见"**威慑**"
means to drive circulation in a gas centrifuge	气体离心机环流驱动法【qìtǐ líxīnjī huánliú qūdòngfǎ】
measurement of nuclear explosion effect parameters	核爆炸效应参数测量【hébàozhà xiàoyìng cānshù cèliáng】
measurement of nuclear fireball parameters	核爆炸火球参数测量【hébàozhà huǒqiú cānshù cèliáng】
measurement technology of nuclear test	核试验测试技术【héshìyàn cèshì jìshù】
mechanical damage induced by X-ray irradiation	X 射线辐照引起的力学损伤【X shèxiàn fúzhào yǐnqǐ de lìxué sǔnshāng】

memorandum	备忘录【bèiwànglù】
metallic fuel	金属燃料【jīnshǔ ránliào】
metallic plutonium	金属钚【jīnshǔbù】
metallic uranium	金属铀【jīnshǔyóu】
methods of tritium production	产氚方法【chǎnchuān fāngfǎ】
militarization of space The deployment of assets (typically satellites) in space for providing information support to military activities. (Modified from: Reference [56], p30) Refer to "**weaponization of space**"	外空军事化【wàikōng jūnshìhuà】 在外空部署设施(通常是卫星)为军事活动提供信息支持。(改自：参考文献[56]，p30) 参见"外空武器化"
military stability	军事稳定性【jūnshì wěndìngxìng】
miniature neutron source reactor (MNSR)	微型中子源反应堆 【wēixíng zhōngzǐyuán fǎnyìngduī】
minimum deterrence Threatening the lowest level of damage necessary to prevent attack, with the fewest number of nuclear weapons possible. (From: Reference [24], p2)	最低核威慑【zuìdī héwēishè】 通过威胁使用最少数量的核武器，产生能够慑止对方攻击所需的最低限度的破坏。(源自：参考文献[24]，p2)
missile accuracy	导弹精度【dǎodàn jīngdù】
Missile Technology Control Regime (MTCR) The MTCR was originally established in 1987 by western countries. It is a regime that aims to restrict the proliferation of systems (except manned air vehicles), equipments and technologies intended for the delivery of weapons of mass destruction (WMD). The MTCR includes the Guidelines and the Equipment and Technology Annex, and it divides controlled items (missiles along with their subsystems and components, production equipments and related technologies) into two	导弹技术控制制度 【dǎodàn jìshù kòngzhì zhìdù】 美国等西方国家 1987 年制定的，旨在防止用于运载大规模杀伤性武器的投掷系统(有人驾驶飞机除外)及有关设备和技术扩散的控制制度。该制度由"准则"和"设备与技术附件"两个文件组成，把限制项目(导弹、分系统、部件，生产设施和有关技术)分成两大类。第一类项目为"最敏感项目"，一般不得转让。第二类项目为军民两用项目，出口

category. Category I items are the most sensitive items, commonly the transfer of them will not be authorized. Category II items are dual-use items, which should be examined and approved case-by-case subject to export license, and be guaranteed not to be used in projects including Category I items. In 1993, member states modified the Guidelines. “Control the transfer of nuclear weapons delivery systems”, in the original version was modified to “control the transfer of weapons of mass destruction (nuclear, biological, chemical weapon) delivery systems”. Up to the end of 2007, the Regime has 34 member states. (Modified from: Reference [1], p410)	时要以许可证方式逐件审批，保证不用于包含第一类项目的系统。1993 年成员国对“准则”进行了修改，把原版中控制“核武器运载系统”的转让改成控制“大规模杀伤性武器(即核、生、化武器)运载系统”的转让。截至 2007 年底，该制度有 34 个成员国。(改自：参考文献[1]，p410)
misuse	滥用【lànyòng】
mixed oxide (MOX)	混合氧化物【hùnhé yǎnghuàwù】
mobile missile	机动导弹【jīdòng dǎodàn】
molecular flow	分子流【fēnzǐliú】
molten salt electrorefining process	熔盐电解精炼流程【róngyán diànjiě jīngliàn liúchéng】
monitoring The means by which information is obtained for verification purposes. (From: Reference [16])	监测【jiāncè】 为核查获取信息的途径。(源自：参考文献[16])
moratorium on nuclear testing	暂停核试验【zàntíng héshìyàn】
multi-fissile body subcritical safety experiment	多裂变体次临界安全实验【duōlièbiàntǐ cìlínjiè ānquán shíyàn】
multiple independently targetable reentry vehicle (MIRV)	分导式多弹头【fēndǎoshì duōdàntóu】

multiplicity of technical protection system	技术防护系统的多重性【jìshù fánghù xìtǒng de duōchóngxìng】
National Ignition Facility (NIF)	国家点火装置【guójiā diǎnhuǒ zhuāngzhì】
national interest	国家利益【guójiā lìyì】
national military strategy The deployment and application of military power to attain national security strategy and national defense strategy objectives. (Modified from: Reference [9], p365)	国家军事战略【guójiā jūnshì zhànlüè】 分配和运用军事力量以实现国家安全战略和国防战略目标。(改自：参考文献[9]，p365)
national security strategy Development, application, and coordination of the instruments of national power to achieve objectives that contribute to national security. In the U.S., it is a formal U.S. government document. (Modified from: Reference [9], p 367)	国家安全战略【guójiā ānquán zhànlüè】 发展、运用和协调各种国家力量手段以实现有助于维护国家安全的目标。在美国，这是一个正式的官方文件。(改自：参考文献[9]，p367)
national strategy	国家战略【guójiā zhànlüè】
national technical means (NTMs) 1 Verification and monitoring technologies or measures owned by a country alone, and information thus collected will be used by itself. NTM is usually used to obtain information or intelligence on relevant activities conducted by other countries. It may also be used for understanding and verifying compliance with treaties or agreements related to arms control by other treaty signatories. (Modified from: Reference [1], p472) 2 NTM refers to nationally owned instruments for surveying a party's compliance with agreement obligations, without intruding onto its territory,	国家技术手段【guójiā jìshù shǒuduàn】 1 一个国家单方面拥有的核查和监测技术或措施，所获信息独家享用，常用于获取其他国家的相关活动的信息或情报。有时，也可用于军备控制条约或协议，以了解和核查其他参约方的遵约情况。(改自：参考文献[1]，p472) 2 在未侵入协议方领土、领空、领海的前提下，国家拥有的用于核查其他协议方是否遵约的手段。来自

airspace or national waters. Information derived from NTM may be used in international verification regimes by a treaty party to question another party's compliance. (From: Reference [19], p198)	NTM 的信息可用于国际核查制度，由条约缔约国向另一方质疑是否遵约。(源自：参考文献[19]，p198)
natural radionuclides	天然放射性核素 【tiānrán fàngshèxìng hésù】
natural uranium	天然铀【tiānrányóu】
naval reactor	海军用反应堆 【hǎijūnyòng fǎnyìngduī】
near-field physical diagnostic To judge nuclear weapons' performance parameters by directly measuring neutrons, γ-rays, and X-rays released from the nuclear reactions. (Modified from: Reference [3], p391)	近区物理诊断【jìnqū wùlǐ zhěnduàn】 直接测量核爆炸过程中伴随着核反应放出的中子、γ射线、X 射线，以判断核武器性能参数。(改自：参考文献[3]，p391)
neutron bomb/enhanced radiation weapon A low-yield hydrogen bomb with a special design utilizing high-energy neutrons as its main destructive element and relatively reducing its shock wave and thermal radiation effects. In a more accurate sense, it is called an "enhanced radiation weapon". (Modified from: Reference [1], p152)	中子弹/增强辐射武器 【zhōngzǐdàn zēngqiáng fúshèwǔqì】 以高能中子为主要毁伤因素，相对减弱冲击波和光辐射效应的一种特殊设计的低威力氢弹。其较确切的名称是增强辐射武器。(改自：参考文献[1]，p152)
neutron generator used in nuclear weapon	核武器用中子发生器 【héwǔqìyòng zhōngzǐ fāshēngqì】
neutrons	中子【zhōngzǐ】
new facility inspection	新设施视察【xīn shèshī shìchá】
new international economic order	国际经济新秩序 【guójì jīngjì xīnzhìxù】
new international political order	国际政治新秩序 【guójì zhèngzhì xīnzhìxù】
new strategic triad	新战略三位一体 【xīn zhànlüè sānwèiyītǐ】

A new U.S. military strategy revealed in the 2002 Nuclear Posture Review, consisting of nuclear and non-nuclear strike forces; passive and active defenses; and a revitalized defense infrastructure. (From: Reference [67]) Refer to "**old nuclear triad**".	美国2002年《核态势评估》报告中提出的一种新的军事战略，由三部分组成：核与非核打击力量；主动的和被动的防御；全新的防御基础设施。(源自：参考文献[67]) 参见"**旧核三位一体**"
new thinking 1 The former Soviet Union President Mikhail Gorbachev's enunciated opinion on the world situation and Soviet Union foreign policy in the 1980s. The main points are: (1) The world is a unity of diversity. (2) Respect the choices of style of life according to people in each country and of the ways of solving their own problems independently. (3) The interest of humanity has priority over that of a class. (4) Nuclear war is a threat to human life and development. And (5) The basis of human common security is respect for independence and sovereignty of other members of the world community. (Modified From: Reference [1], p34; [64])	**新思维【xīnsīwéi】** 1 20世纪80年代中期苏联领导人戈尔巴乔夫对当时世界的看法以及关于苏联外交政策的观点，主要内容为：(1)世界是一个多样性的统一体；(2)充分尊重各国人民按照自己的选择而生活并独立自主地解决自身的问题；(3)全人类的利益高于阶级利益；(4)战争威胁着人类的生存与发展；(5)全人类普遍安全的唯一原则基础是尊重主权。(改自:参考文献[1]，p34；[64])
2 The term used to characterize distinctive elements in Soviet foreign policy thinking developed under the leadership of President Mikhail Gorbachev in the latter half of the 1980s. The main propositions in new thinking included: (1) the relationship between capitalist and socialist states was not zero-sum; (2) common human interests should take priority over class-based interests; (3) military parity with the U.S. was not necessary for Soviet security, and non-offensive	2 该术语用以描述20世纪80年代中后期在戈尔巴乔夫总统领导下而发展的苏联外交政策思维的特性。新思维的主要观点包括：(1)资本主义和社会主义之间不是"零和"关系；(2)共同的人类利益高于阶级利益；(3)与美国的军事均衡对苏联的安全不是必需的，非攻击性的防御战略应优于进攻战略；(4)军事力量主要用于防止冲突，而不是在战争

defensive strategies were preferable to offensive strategies; (4) the main purpose of military power was to prevent conflict, rather than to defeat an adversary in a war. Some of the manifestations of new thinking included certain unilateral disarmament measures, reductions in the size of certain military forces, and a strong commitment to bilateral and multilateral confidence building and arms control measures. (From: Reference [57], p117-129; [58])	中打败对手。新思维的某些表现形式包括单边裁军措施、削减军事力量、承诺单边和多边的信任建立及裁军措施。(源自：参考文献[57]，p117-129；[58])
new triad Refer to **"new strategic triad"**.	新三位一体【xīn sānwèiyītǐ】 参见"新战略三位一体"
no-first-use of nuclear weapons	不首先使用核武器 【bù shǒuxiān shǐyòng héwǔqì】
nonaligned movement	不结盟运动【bùjiéméng yùndòng】
non-application of IAEA safeguards	不实施国际原子能机构的保障监督 【bùshíshī guójì yuánzǐnéng jīgòu de bǎozhàng jiāndū】
non-compliance	不遵约【bùzūnyuē】
non-nuclear weapon state (NNWS)	无核武器国家【wú héwǔqì guójiā】
non-proliferation	不扩散【bùkuòsàn】
(North South) Joint Declaration on the Denuclearization of the Korean Peninsula	关于朝鲜半岛无核化共同宣言 【guānyú cháoxiǎn bàndǎo wúhéhuà gòngtóng xuānyán】
NPT Review Conferences	《不扩散核武器条约》审议会 【bùkuòsàn héwǔqì tiáoyuē shěnyìhuì】
nuclear airburst	空中核爆炸【kōngzhōng hébàozhà】
nuclear artillery projectile	核炮弹【hépàodàn】
nuclear blackmail	核讹诈【hé'ézhà】
nuclear bomb	核炸弹【hézhàdàn】

nuclear campaign A series of related military operations using nuclear weapons aimed at accomplishing a strategic or operational objective within a given time and space. (Modified from: Reference [9], p76)	核战役【hézhànyì】 在一定时间和区域内为实现战役或战略目标所采取的一系列使用核武器的相关军事行动。(改自：参考文献[9]，p76)
nuclear counterattack	核反击【héfǎnjī】
nuclear decay	核衰变【héshuāibiàn】
nuclear depth bomb	核深水炸弹【hé shēnshuǐ zhàdàn】
nuclear deterrence A strategy of preventing a nuclear attack by threatening the perceived or potential enemy with unacceptable damage by nuclear retaliation. (From: Reference [6], p177) Note: In principle, nuclear deterrence could be used to deter not only nuclear attacks but also attacks with conventional forces, attacks with chemical or biological weapons, or even assaults on vital national interests by nonmilitary means. (From: Reference [7], p14-15)	核威慑【héwēishè】 以给觉察到的或潜在的敌人造成无法承受的毁伤的核报复相威胁，从而防止敌人实施核打击的战略。(源自：参考文献[6]，p177) 注：原则上，核威慑不仅仅可以用来阻止核攻击，而且也可以用来阻止常规力量、化学或生物武器的攻击，甚至用来阻止由非军事手段使至关重要的国家利益遭受损害的攻击。(源自：参考文献[7]，p14-15)
nuclear doctrine The fundamental principles governing the conditions under which and the modalities of how nuclear weapons are to be used in support of national objectives. (Modified from: Reference [9])	核学说【héxuéshuō】 为支持国家战略目标而规定在何种情形下以何种方式使用核武器的基本原则。(改自：参考文献[9])
nuclear earth penetrator	核钻地弹【hézuāndìdàn】
nuclear electromagnetic pulse (NEMP)	核电磁脉冲【hédiàncí màichōng】
nuclear energy level	核能级【hénéngjí】
nuclear explosion The process of producing explosive	核爆炸【hébàozhà】 利用能自持进行的原子核裂变或/

effects and potentially huge casualties and damage by huge energy instantaneously released from selfsustaining nuclear fission or/and fusion. (Modified from: Reference [3], p394) Note: A nuclear explosion is a self-sustaining fission chain reaction (or fission-fusion reaction) in a material that is disrupted in the process, with the exception of inertial-confinement fusion systems for obtaining energy from pure nuclear fusion. A nuclear reactor, even a pulsed nuclear reactor in which the fission process is terminated by thermal expansion of solid material, is not a nuclear explosion. (Modified from: Reference [59], p14-15)	和聚变反应瞬时释放的巨大能量，产生爆炸作用和可能造成巨大杀伤破坏效应的过程。(改自：参考文献[3]，p394) 注：核爆炸指由于在材料中发生自持裂变链式反应或裂变－聚变反应而导致材料解体(从纯粹的核聚变中获得能量的惯性约束聚变系统除外)。核反应堆，即使是裂变过程由于固体材料热膨胀而终止的脉冲核反应堆，也不属于核爆炸。(改自：参考文献[59]，p14-15)
nuclear explosion debris fractionation	核爆炸碎片的分凝 【hébàozhà suìpiàn de fēnníng】
nuclear-explosion-driven microwave weapon A nuclear explosive with special characteristics coupled with a special microwave generator that can disturb or destroy enemies' communication system or electronic components of weapons by high-power microwaves. It is one of the proposed third generation nuclear weapons. (Modified from: Reference [2], p176)	核爆激励高功率微波武器 【hébào jīlì gāogōnglǜ wēibō wǔqì】 一种具有特殊性能的核爆炸装置，它通过与微波发生器耦合的方式，产生以高功率微波干扰或毁坏敌方通信系统或武器的电子部件。又称核爆驱动电磁脉冲弹。它是提议中第三代核武器的一种。(改自：参考文献[2]，p176)
nuclear explosion effects	核爆炸效应【hébàozhà xiàoyìng】
nuclear explosion fireball	核爆炸火球【hébàozhà huǒqiú】
nuclear-explosion-level prompt radiation simulation source	核爆炸级瞬时辐射模拟源 【hébàozhàjí shùnshí fúshè mónǐ yuán】
nuclear explosion shock wave	核爆炸冲击波【hébàozhà chōngjībō】

E I C

nuclear explosive device A fission or thermonuclear device capable of producing a nuclear explosion. (Modified from: Reference [3], p379)	**核爆炸装置【hébàozhà zhuāngzhì】** 具有核爆炸功能的裂变装置或热核装置。(改自：参考文献[3]，p379)
nuclear-explosive material (NEM) Any mixture of nuclear-explosive and other nuclides that can be made to support a chain reaction when present in suitable quantity, purity, and geometry is called “nuclear-explosive material” (NEM). (From: Reference [11], p221)	**核爆材料【hébào cáiliào】** 以适当的数量、纯度和构型存在时，能用以支持链式反应的核炸药和其他核素的混合物。(源自：参考文献[11]，p221)
nuclear export control Control of commercial export, gifts to and exhibitions in foreign countries or regions, as well as scientific and technological cooperation with and assistance to foreign countries or regions that involve nuclear materials, nuclear equipment, non-nuclear materials used for reactors and other items as well as their related technologies. (Modified from: Reference [25])	**核出口控制【héchūkǒu kòngzhì】** 对核材料、核设备和反应堆用非核材料等物项及其相关技术的贸易性出口及对外赠送、展览、科技合作和援助进行控制。(改自：参考文献[25])
nuclear first strike 1 The launching of an initial nuclear attack before one’s opponent is able to use any strategic weapon. First strike is a nuclear attack carried out at such a devastatingly high level of destruction as to nullify an enemy’s capability to launch a major counterstrike. (From: Reference [6], p72) 2 An initial attack on an opponent's strategic nuclear forces. Such an attack may be undertaken in an attempt to destroy an enemy's retaliatory (second-strike) capability. (From: Reference [8])	**第一次核打击【dìyīcì hédǎjī】** 1 在对手能够使用任何战略武器之前率先发动核攻击。首次打击是给对手造成极大的破坏致使其失去发起有效反击能力的核进攻。(源自：参考文献[6]，p72) 2 对敌方战略核力量的首次打击。这种打击可用于试图摧毁敌方的报复(第二次打击)能力。(源自：参考文献[8])

nuclear fission	核裂变【hélièbiàn】
nuclear football A popular name of a portable briefcase or package that contains instructions and codes for the president to authorize the use of strategic nuclear weapons. (Modified from: Reference[2], p203)	核黑匣子【hé hēixiázi】 装有总统用来授权使用战略核武器的指令和密码的便携手提箱或手提包的俗称。(改自：参考文献[2]，p203)
nuclear forces	核武装力量【héwǔzhuāng lìliàng】
nuclear fuel	核燃料【héránliào】
nuclear fuel cycle A system of nuclear installations and activities interconnected by streams of nuclear material. The characteristics of the fuel cycle may vary widely from State to State, from a single reactor supplied from abroad with fuel, to a fully developed system. (From: Reference [4], 4.30)	核燃料循环【héránliào xúnhuán】 由与核材料物流相关的核设施及核活动组成的系统。从由国外提供带燃料的单个反应堆，到一整套完善系统，不同国家之间燃料循环的特点可能存在很大差异。(源自：参考文献[4]，4.30)
nuclear fuel reprocessing	核燃料后处理【héránliào hòuchǔlǐ】
nuclear hardening	抗核加固【kànghé jiāgù】
nuclear heating reactor	供热反应堆【gōngrè fǎnyìngduī】
nuclear high altitude burst	高空核爆炸【gāokōng hébàozhà】
nuclear land (water) surface burst	地(水)面核爆炸 【dìshuǐmiàn hébàozhà】
nuclear loss Loss of nuclear material due to its transformation into other element(s) or isotope(s) as a result of nuclear reactions. Nuclear loss also includes burn up of nuclear material in a reactor and decay (e.g. of Pu-241) during storage. (From: Reference [4], 6.22)	核损耗【hésǔnhào】 指由于核反应使核材料转变成其他元素或同位素而造成的核材料损耗。核损耗还包括核材料在反应堆中燃烧所造成的损耗以及存储期间衰变所造成的损耗(例如钚-241 的衰变)。(源自：参考文献[4]，6.22)
nuclear material	核材料【hécáiliào】

nuclear material accountancy The practice of nuclear material accounting as implemented by the facility operator and the State system of accounting for and control of nuclear material (SSAC), inter alia, to satisfy the requirements in the safeguards agreement between the IAEA and the State (or group of States); and as implemented by the IAEA, inter alia, to independently verify the correctness of the nuclear material accounting information in the facility records and the reports provided by the SSAC to the IAEA. (From: Reference [4], 6.2)	**核材料衡算活动** 【hé cá ilià hé ngsuà huđòg 】 设施运行者和国家核材料衡算和控制系统所采取的衡算核材料的行动，尤其是为满足 IAEA 和该国(或国家集团)之间的保障监督协议的要求，也包括 IAEA 所采取的类似行动，尤其是为独立核查国家核材料衡算和控制系统(SSAC)向 IAEA 所提供的设施纪录和报告中核材料衡算信息的正确性。(源自：参考文献[4]，6.2)
nuclear material incident	**核材料意外事件** 【hécáiliào yìwài shìjiàn】
nuclear matter	**核物质**【héwùzhì】
nuclear missile reentry vehicle 1 A missile reentry vehicle equipped with a nuclear warhead. (From: Reference [3], p96) 2 reentry vehicle (RV) — The part of a space vehicle designed to re-enter the earth's atmosphere. (From: Reference [9], p456) 3 reentry vehicle (RV) — A nuclear warhead on a ballistic missile specially designed to reenter the earth's atmosphere in the terminal portion of the missile's trajectory. (From: Reference [8]) Note: The term "reentry body" is the less-common equivalent of "reentry vehicle".	**核导弹弹头**【hédǎodàn dàntóu】 1 装有核战斗部的导弹再入飞行器。(源自：参考文献[3]，p96) 2 再入飞行器——设计为再入地球大气层的空间飞行器部件。(源自：参考文献[9]，p456) 3 再入飞行器(或(再入)弹头)——在导弹的弹道终端能再入地球大气层的弹道导弹上的核战斗部。(源自：参考文献[8]) 注：“再入飞行器”的一种非常用名称是“再入体”。
nuclear operation plan	**核作战计划**【hézuòzhàn jìhuà】
nuclear primacy The condition whereby one state holds	**核优势**【héyōushì】 一个核国家的核武器拥有明显的质

a clear qualitative and quantitative ability to prevent or render ineffective a rival's retaliatory (second) strike capability. (Modified from: Reference [22])	量和数量上的优势足以阻止或摧毁对手的报复性(第二次)打击能力的状态。(改自：参考文献[22])
Note: In another view, "The ability to destroy all of an adversary's nuclear forces, eliminating the possibility of a retaliatory strike, is known as a first-strike capability, or nuclear primacy." (From: Reference [22])	注：另一种观点是，"摧毁对手所有核力量、消除报复性打击可能性的能力，被认为是一种第一次打击能力或核优势"。(源自：参考文献[22])
nuclear reaction	**核反应【héfǎnyìng】**
nuclear-related dual-use item An item which has a technical use in both nuclear and non-nuclear applications, and may be subject to certain conditions of supply because such items could make a major contribution to a nuclear explosive activity. (Modified from: Reference [4], 5.34)	**核相关两用物项** **【hé xiāngguān liǎngyòng wùxiàng】** 指一种在核和非核领域都有技术用途的物项，提供这种物项时要遵守一定条件，因为这种物项可能为核爆炸活动提供很大的帮助。(改自：参考文献[4]，5.34)
Nuclear Safety Convention	**核安全公约【hé'ānquán gōngyuē】**
nuclear second strike Retaliatory nuclear attack following an enemy's first nuclear attack. (Modified from: Reference [2], p62)	**第二次核打击【dì'èrcì hédǎjī】** 对敌方第一次核袭击的报复性核打击。(改自：参考文献[2]，p62)
nuclear strategy Strategy of planning and guiding the development and employment of nuclear force. (From: Reference [1], p112)	**核战略【hézhànlüè】** 筹划和指导核力量发展与运用的方略。(源自：参考文献[1]，p112)
nuclear strike	**核打击【hédǎjī】**
Nuclear Suppliers Group (NSG) A group of nuclear supplier countries which seeks to contribute to the non-proliferation of nuclear weapons through the implementation of Guide-	**核供应国集团【hégōngyìngguó jítuán】** 通过执行核(和涉及核)出口准则而防止核武器扩散的核供应国家。各参与国通过其国家法律和惯例来执

lines for nuclear exports and nuclear related exports. The NSG Guidelines are implemented by each Participating Government in accordance with its national laws and practices. Decisions on export applications are taken at the national level in accordance with national export licensing requirements. (From: Reference [47])	行核供应国集团的准则。出口申请由国家层面决定，并符合国家出口许可规定。(源自：参考文献[47])
Nuclear Suppliers Group Guidelines	**核供应国集团准则** 【hégōngyìngguó jítuán zhǔnzé】
nuclear test	**核试验**【héshìyàn】
nuclear test site	**核试验场**【héshìyànchǎng】
nuclear threat	**核威胁**【héwēixié】
nuclear threshold state (NTS)	**核门槛国家**【héménkǎn guójiā】
nuclear underground (or underwater) burst	**地(水)下核爆炸** 【dìshuǐxià hébàozhà】
nuclear war	**核战争**【hézhànzhēng】
nuclear warfighting capability In nuclear strategy, having the capability to use nuclear weapons to fight a war, and not just to deter the outbreak of nuclear war. (Modified from: Reference [48])	**核战能力**【hézhàn nénglì】 在核战略中，具有使用核武器进行战争的能力，而不仅限于慑止核战争爆发的能力。(改自：参考文献[48])
nuclear warhead The part of a nuclear weapon whose function is to destroy or damage targets. It mainly consists of a nuclear explosive device, arming, fuzing and firing system, and other functional parts or relevant structures. In Chinese writings in the arms control field, the nuclear warhead is often called 【hédàntóu】(核弹头). (Modified from: Reference [3], p404) Note: The warhead is that part of a	**核战斗部**【hézhàndòubù】 核武器中用来毁伤目标的部分。主要由核爆炸装置、引爆控制系统、其他功能部件和相应的结构部件等组成。在中国军备控制领域常把核战斗部称为核弹头。(改自：参考文献[3]，p404) 注：战斗部——导弹、炮弹、鱼雷、

missile, projectile, torpedo, rocket, or other munition which contains either the nuclear or thermonuclear system, high explosive system, chemical or biological agents or inert materials intended to inflict damage. (From: Reference [5], p15)	火箭或其他武器的毁伤目标的部分，它含有核或热核系统、高能炸药系统、生物或化学制剂、或惰性材料。(源自：参考文献[5]，p15)
nuclear weapon 1 Weapon assembly that is capable of producing an explosion and massive injury and destruction by the sudden release of energy instantaneously released from self-sustaining nuclear fission and/or fusion. From the generalized point of view, it refers to a nuclear weapon system with a warfighting capability including the delivery or launch system. (Modified from: Reference [3], p394)	**核武器【héwǔqì】** 1 利用能自持进行的原子核裂变和(或)聚变反应瞬时释放的巨大能量，产生爆炸作用，并具有大规模毁伤破坏效应的武器。从广义上说它是指包括投掷或发射系统在内的具有作战能力的核武器系统。(改自：参考文献[3]，p394)
2 NATO definition —— A complete assembly (i.e. implosion type, gun type or thermonuclear type) in its intended ultimate configuration which, upon completion of the prescribed arming, fusing and firing sequence, is capable of producing the intended nuclear reaction and release of energy. Also called "atomic weapon". (From: Reference [49], p11)	2 北约定义——根据预期设计构造，在完成指定的引爆控制序列后，能够产生预期的核反应并释放出核能的完整装置(如内爆型、枪型或热核型)。也被称为"原子武器"。(源自：参考文献[49]，p11)
3 Russian definition —— Nuclear Weapons in the Armed Forces of the Russian Federation include an aggregate of armaments including nuclear charges, nuclear ammunition, means of their delivery to the target and control means. (From: Reference [29], p21)	3 俄罗斯定义——俄罗斯联邦军队的核武器是指包括核装料、核战斗部、运载工具和控制系统在内的武器系统。(源自：参考文献[29]，p21)
4 A device that releases nuclear energy in an explosive manner as the result of nuclear chain reactions involving the	4 使原子核产生裂变或聚变链式反应(或兼而有之)，以爆炸方式释放

E-C

fission or fusion, or both, of atomic nuclei. (From: Reference [8])	核能的装置。(源自：参考文献[8])
nuclear weapon accidents	核武器事故【héwǔqì shìgù】
nuclear weapon miniaturization	核武器小型化【héwǔqì xiǎoxínghuà】
nuclear weapon physics	核武器物理【héwǔqì wùlǐ】
nuclear weapon safety In maintenance and use of nuclear weapons, the capability to avoid an accident involving personnel, facilities and installations due to misuse or from gradual deterioration or a sudden fault in equipment or weapons. (Modified from: Reference [2], p217)	核武器安全性【héwǔqì ānquánxìng】 在正常的维护或使用核武器中，防止因设备或武器的误操作、逐步退化或意外故障等原因发生人员、设备和设施的事故的能力。(改自：参考文献[2]，p217)
nuclear weapon security The capability of a nuclear weapon and its surrounding equipment and personnel to prevent any unauthorized use. (Modified from: Reference [2], p217)	核武器保安性【héwǔqì bǎo'ānxìng】 核武器及其相关的设备和人员能抵制任何非授权的使用的能力。(改自：参考文献[2]，p217)
nuclear weapon state (NWS)	核武器国家【héwǔqì guójiā】
nuclear weapons stockpile	核武器库存【héwǔqì kùcún】
nuclear weapons surety The materiel, personnel, and procedures that contribute to the safety, security, reliability, and control of nuclear weapons, thus assuring no nuclear accidents, incidents, unauthorized use, or degradation in performance. (From: Reference [60])	核武器确信性 【héwǔqì quèxìnxìng】 使用能提高核武器安全性、保安性、可靠性和可控性的材料、人员和程序，以确保核武器在使用过程中不发生核事故、故障、非授权使用或功能退化。(源自：参考文献[60])
nuclear winter	核冬天【hédōngtiān】
nucleon	核子【hézǐ】
nuclide	核素【hésù】
ocean surveillance satellite	海洋监视卫星 【hǎiyáng jiānshì wèixīng】

offensive strategy A strategy that aims to carry military operations to the enemy by closing with and destroying enemy forces, seizing territory and vital resources. Its focus is on seizing, retaining, and exploiting the initiative. (From: Reference [61], p3-27)	进攻性战略【jìngōngxìng zhànlüè】 为接近并摧毁敌方军事力量以及夺取疆土和重要资源而对敌方采取的军事行动。它致力于抢占、保持和发挥主动权。(源自：参考文献[61]，p3-27)
off-load refuelled power reactor	停堆换料动力堆 【tíngduī huànliào dònglìduī】
old nuclear triad The three legs of the U.S. strategic nuclear force: submarine-launched ballistic missiles (SLBMs), land based intercontinental ballistic missiles (ICBMs) and long-range bombers. (From: Reference [72]) Refer to **"new strategic triad"**	旧核三位一体【jiù hé sānweìyītǐ】 美国战略核力量的三个支柱：潜射弹道导弹(SLBMs)；陆基洲际弹道导弹(ICBMs)；远程轰炸机。(源自：参考文献[72]) 参见"新战略三位一体"
once-through nuclear fuel cycle	一次通过式核燃料循环 【yīcì tōngguòshì héránliào xúnhuán】
one-point safety of a nuclear weapon Safety performance of a nuclear weapon when any one point of the high explosive is detonated in abnormal situations (by impact, projectile, etc). The U.S. military standard is that the probability of releasing more than 1.8 kg TNT equivalent fission energy when any point of the explosive is ignited is less than one per million in any accident. (Modified from: Reference [2], p223)	核武器一点安全 【héwǔqì yīdiǎn ānquán】 核武器在异常环境(撞击或枪击)下武器中炸药任何一点起爆时所具有的安全性能。美国军用标准为：在任何事故中，炸药任何一点起爆时所产生的裂变能在 1.8 千克梯恩梯当量以上的概率小于百万分之一。(改自：参考文献[2]，p223)
on-load refuelled power reactor	不停堆换料动力堆 【bùtíngduī huànliào dònglìduī】
on-site inspection (OSI) The verification method carried out by personnel or apparatus on the selected site. The 13 types of inspection are	现场视察【xiànchǎng shìchá】 在被探测现场利用人员或仪器收集信息的视察方式。《美苏关于削减

E I C

defined in the START I treaty. Inspections are carried out by designated inspectors to verify that particular activities prohibited by an arms limitation agreement are not performed, to check that particular activities prescribed by an arms limitation agreement are implemented, or to examine the nature of a suspicious event. (Modified from:Reference [16], p231)	和限制进攻性战略武器条约》规定了 13 种现场视察方式。视察由指派的视察员执行，旨在核实没有进行军备限制协议所禁止的活动，确认执行了军备限制协议所规定的活动，或调查可疑事件的真相。(改自：参考文献[16]，p231)
Open Skies Treaty	开放天空条约 【kāifàng tiānkōng tiáoyuē】
operating records	运行记录【yùnxíng jìlù】
operational capability	实战能力【shízhàn nénglì】
operational characteristics of nuclear weapon	核武器战术技术性能 【héwǔqì zhànshù jìshù xìngnéng】
operationally deployed warhead	实战部署的弹头 【shízhàn bùshǔ de dàntóu】
operations research and analysis of nuclear weapon employment	核武器运用的运筹分析 【héwǔqì yùnyòng de yùnchóu fēnxī】
Organization for Security and Cooperation in Europe (OSCE)	欧洲安全与合作组织 【ōuzhōu ānquán yǔ hézuò zǔzhī】
overall design of nuclear weapon	核武器总体设计 【héwǔqì zǒngtǐ shèjì】
passive gamma-ray detection A rapid and non-destructive detection of fissionable materials and equipments containing fissionable material through detecting characteristic gamma-rays emitted from decay of such fissionable material. (From: Reference [1], p495)	无源γ射线探测 【wúyuán γ shèxiàn tàncè】 通过测量裂变材料衰变时产生的特征γ射线，对裂变材料及含裂变材料的装置进行快速、无损探测的方法。(源自：参考文献[1]，p495)
passive neutron detection A method of rapid non-destructive detection of fissionable material or devices containing fissionable materials	无源中子探测 【wúyuán zhōngzǐ tàncè】 通过探测裂变材料的自发中子而对裂变材料或含裂变材料的装置进行

by detecting neutrons spontaneously emitted from such fissionable material. (From: Reference [1], p496)	快速无损探测的方法。(源自：参考文献[1]，p495)
passive seal Refer to "**seal**"	无源封记【wúyuán fēngjì】 参见"封记"
passive tag Refer to "**tag**"	无源标签【wúyuán biāoqiān】 参见"标签"
path-length fuze of nuclear weapon	核武器路程长度引信 【héwǔqì lùchéng chángdù yǐnxìn】
payload	有效载荷【yǒuxiào zàihè】
peaceful nuclear explosions	和平核爆炸【hépíng hébàozhà】
peaceful use of nuclear explosion	和平利用核爆炸 【hépíng lìyòng hébàozhà】
pellet	芯块【xīnkuài】
penetration ability of nuclear weapon	核武器突防能力 【héwǔqì tūfáng nénglì】
penetration aids of nuclear missiles	核导弹的突防装置 【hédǎodàn de tūfáng zhuāngzhì】
perimeter portal continuous monitoring	设施周边与进出口连续监测 【shèshī zhōubiān yǔ jìnchūkǒu liánxù jiāncè】
permanent radiation damage in electronics	电子系统的永久性辐射损伤 【diànzǐ xìtǒng de yǒngjiǔxìng fúshè sǔnshāng】
permeability of barrier	分离膜的渗透性 【fēnlímó de shèntòuxìng】
permissive action link (PAL) A device included in or attached to a nuclear weapon system to preclude arming and/or launching until the insertion of a prescribed discrete code. (From: Reference[9], p412) Refer to "**safing device of nuclear weapon**"	密码锁(亦称启动连接装置) 【mìmǎsuǒ yìchēng qǐdòng liánjiē zhuāngzhì】 一种安装或附加在核武器系统上的装置，用于在输入预定的离散密码前，防止解除保险和(或)发射。(源自：参考文献[9]，p412) 参见"核武器保险装置"

physical barrier for protected sections	保护区实体屏障 【bǎohùqū shítǐ píngzhàng】
physical diagnostic measurement in nuclear test	核试验的物理诊断测量 【héshìyàn de wùlǐzhěnduàn cèliáng】
physical inventory The sum of all the measured or derived estimates of batch quantities of nuclear material on hand at a given time within a material balance area, obtained in accordance with specified procedures. (Modified from: Reference [15], para113; [4], 6.41)	实物存量【shíwù cúnliàng】 某一给定时刻，在特定核材料平衡区内，按照规定程序测量或估算所得到的所有批量的核材料总和。(改自：参考文献[15]，para113；[4]，6.41)
physical inventory-taking of nuclear material The activities carried out to determine physical inventory. (Modified from: Reference [15], para113; [4], 6.41)	核材料实物盘存 【hécáiliào shíwù páncún】 为确定核材料实物存量而采取的行动。(改自：参考文献[15]，para113；[4]，6.41)
physical-protection authorization of nuclear material	核材料实体保护授权 【hécáiliào shítǐ bǎohù shòuquán】
physical-protection design basis threats	实体保护设计基准威胁 【shítǐ bǎohù shèjì jīzhǔn wēixié】
physical-protection emergency response	实体保护应急响应 【shítǐ bǎohù yìngjí xiǎngyìng】
physical-protection for nuclear material Establishing a security protection system for extant buildings and vehicles (relating to storage or transportation processes) with nuclear material, so as to safeguard nuclear material. (From: Reference [2], p186)	核材料实体保护 【hécáiliào shítǐ bǎohù】 对存有核材料的建筑物和车辆(涉及储存和运输过程)等建立安全防范系统，以实施对核材料的保障监督。(源自：参考文献[2]，p186)
physical-protection levels of nuclear material	核材料实体保护等级 【hécáiliào shítǐ bǎohù děngjí】
physical-protection organization	实体保护组织机构 【shítǐ bǎohù zǔzhī jīgòu】
physical-protection recommendations	实体保护建议【shítǐ bǎohù jiànyì】

physical-protection system-failure criterion	实体保护系统失效判断准则【shítǐ bǎohù xìtǒng shīxiào pànduàn zhǔnzé】
physical-simulation of nuclear explosion	核爆炸物理模拟【hébàozhà wùlǐ mónǐ】
physics package The primary and secondary of a nuclear weapon are housed inside a radiation case; the completed assembly is called the "physics package." (From: Reference [11], p91)	物理包【wùlǐbāo】 核武器中封装在辐射壳内的初级和次级部件的完整的组装件。(源自：参考文献[11]，p91)
pit The sphere or shell of nuclear explosive material at the center of an implosion device, usually clad with beryllium or another metal. (Modified from: Reference [11], p90)	弹芯【dànxīn】 安置在内爆装置中心、通常有铍或其他金属包层的核炸药材料球体或壳体。(改自：参考文献[11]，p90)
plutonium	钚【bù】
plutonium alloy	钚合金【bùhéjīn】
plutonium decontamination cycle	钚净化循环【bù jìnghuà xúnhuán】
plutonium dioxide	二氧化钚【èryǎnghuàbù】
plutonium recycling A process of reusing in nuclear reactors the plutonium extracted from spent fuel. (From: Reference [2], p22) Note: In the DUPIC process, spent LWR fuel rods are directly used as fuel for CANDU-type heavy-water power reactors, with only mechanical modifications and not chemical reprocessing. (From: Reference [32], p25-40)	钚再循环【bù zàixúnhuán】 将从乏燃料中回收得到的钚在反应堆内再使用的过程。(源自：参考文献[2]，p22) 注：在 DUPIC 过程中，轻水堆的乏燃料棒只需机械处理而不需化学后处理即可直接作为 CANDU 型重水动力堆的燃料。(源自：参考文献[32]，p25-40)
point sample An environmental sample taken in one particular area to characterize one source of released material which can	点样品【diǎn yàngpǐn】 在一个特定地区环境为确定能够在接近泄漏点临近地区发现泄漏物质

E I C

be found in a contiguous area adjacent to a release point. (From: Reference [4], 9.5)	的源的特征而采集的样品。(源自：参考文献[4]，9.5)
point target	点目标【diǎn mùbiāo】
post-exercise dispersal inspection	演习后疏散视察【yǎnxíhòu shūsàn shìchá】
power reactor	动力堆【dònglìduī】
powered phase	主动段【zhǔdòngduàn】
predetonation in fission explosion	裂变爆炸过早点火【lièbiàn bàozhà guòzǎo diǎnhuǒ】
preemptive strike	先发制人打击【xiānfāzhìrén dǎjī】
preset burst depth of nuclear weapon	核武器装订爆深【héwǔqì zhuāngdìng bàoshēn】
preset burst height of nuclear weapon	核武器装订爆高【héwǔqì zhuāngdìng bàogāo】
pressurized water reactor (PWR)	压水堆【yāshuǐduī】
principal nuclear facility	重要核设施【zhòngyào héshèshī】
Principled Declaration on Refraining from the Threat or Use of Force in Their International Relations	关于国际关系中不得进行武力威胁或使用武力的原则宣言【guānyú guójìguānxì zhōng bùdé jìnxíng wǔlì wēixié huò shǐyòng wǔlì de yuánzé xuānyán】
processing of radioactive liquid waste	放射性废液处理【fàngshèxìng fèiyè chǔlǐ】
production of uranium hexafluoride by fluorination of uranium tetrafluoride	四氟化铀氟化生产六氟化铀【sìfúhuàyóu fúhuà shēngchǎn liùfúhuàyóu】
production reactor	生产堆【shēngchǎnduī】
prohibition of the production of fissile material for nuclear weapon	禁止为核武器生产易裂变材料【jìnzhǐ wèi héwǔqì shēngchǎn yìlièbiàn cáiliào】
project and supply agreement	项目和供应协定【xiàngmù hé gōngyìng xiédìng】

projection of nuclear weapon	核武器投射【héwǔqì tóushè】
propagation of nuclear electromagnetic pulse	核电磁脉冲的传播 【hédiàncímàichōng de chuánbō】
protection from nuclear electromagnetic pulse	核电磁脉冲的防护 【hédiàncí màichōng de fánghù】
protection of nuclear weapon	核武器的防护 【héwǔqì de fánghù】
protocol	议定书【yìdìngshū】
Protocol to the Treaty Between the United States of America and the Union of Soviet Socialist Republics on the Reduction and Limitation of Strategic Offensive Arms	美苏关于削减和限制进攻性战略武器条约议定书 【měi sū guānyú xuējiǎn hé xiànzhì jìngōngxìng zhànlüèwǔqì tiáoyuē yìdìngshū】
proton	质子【zhìzǐ】
PUREX (Plutonium Uranium Recovery by Extraction) process	普雷克斯流程【pǔléikèsī liúchéng】 (钚铀的萃取回收流程)
pyrochemical processing	高温化学处理【gāowēn huàxué chǔlǐ】
pyrometallurgical processing	高温冶金处理【gāowēn yějīn chǔlǐ】
radar fuze of nuclear weapon	核武器雷达引信【héwǔqì léidá yǐnxìn】
radiation	辐射【fúshè】
radiation-hardened electronic components	辐射加固的电子器件 【fúshè jiāgù de diànzǐ qìjiàn】
radioactive aerosol of nuclear explosion	核爆炸产生的放射性气溶胶 【hébàozhà chǎnshēng de fàngshèxìng qìróngjiāo】
radioactive cloud	放射性烟云【fàngshèxìng yānyún】
radioactive contamination	放射性沾染【fàngshèxìng zhānrǎn】
radioactive fallout	放射性沉降【fàngshèxìng chénjiàng】
radioactive gas sampling and detecting	放射性气体取样与探测 【fàngshèxìng qìtǐ qǔyàng yǔ tàncè】

radioactive nuclide from nuclear explosion	核爆炸产生的放射性核素【hébàozhà chǎnshēng de fàngshèxìng hésù】
radioactive waste	放射性废物【fàngshèxìng fèiwù】
radioactive waste disposal	放射性废物处置【fàngshèxìng fèiwù chǔzhì】
radioactivity	放射性活度【fàngshèxìng huódù】
radiochemical diagnostic of nuclear test	核试验放射化学诊断【héshìyàn fàngshèhuàxué zhěnduàn】
radioisotope	放射性同位素【fàngshèxìng tóngwèisù】
radiological dispersal device (RDD) Refer to **“dirty bomb”**	放射性物质散布装置【fàngshèxìng wùzhì sànbù zhuāngzhì】 参见“脏弹”
radionuclide monitoring A method for monitoring nuclear related activity through collecting, analyzing, and measuring different kinds of radionuclides. (Modified from: Reference [1], p486)	放射性核素监测【fàngshèxìng hésù jiāncè】 通过收集、分析、测量各种放射性核素，以达到监测相关核活动目的的方法。(改自：参考文献[1]，p486)
random inspection An inspection performed at a facility or a location outside facilities on a date chosen randomly. (From: Reference [4], 11.8)	随机视察【suíjī shìchá】 在一个随机选定的日期对一处设施或设施外的一处场地进行的视察。(源自：参考文献[4]，11.8)
random sampling The process of selecting samples in such a manner that all items in a population have the same probability of being selected. (From: Reference [4], 7.8)	随机取样【suíjī qǔyàng】 所涉群体内的所有物项有相同被选概率的取样方式。(源自：参考文献[4]，7.8)
range of nuclear missiles	核导弹射程【hédǎodàn shèchéng】
reactor	反应堆【fǎnyìngduī】
reactor-grade plutonium Plutonium containing more than 18% Pu-240. (Modified from: Reference [2], p93)	反应堆级钚【fǎnyìngduījí bù】 通常指钚-240 含量大于 18%的钚。(改自：参考文献[2]，p93)

real cascade	实际级联【shíjì jílián】
real-time monitoring Monitoring information which has been delayed only by the time required for electronic communication, implying that there are no noticeable delays. (Modified from: Reference [9], p451)	实时监测【shíshí jiāncè】 除了电子通信所必需的时间外，没有显著延迟地对数据或信息进行的及时的监测。(改自：参考文献[9]，p451)
redox process	雷道克斯流程【léidàokèsī liúchéng】
reduced residual radioactivity weapon (RRRW)	弱剩余放射性武器(3R 弹) 【ruò shèngyú fàngshèxìng wǔqì 3Rdàn】
reduced yield nuclear test	减威力核试验【jiǎnwēilì héshìyàn】
reduction	削减【xuējiǎn】
reentry phase	再入段【zàirùduàn】
reentry telemetry for nuclear reentry vehicle	核弹头再入遥测 【hédàntóu zàirù yáocè】
reference material	参考物质【cānkǎo wùzhì】
reflector (tamper) layer in atomic bomb	原子弹反射层(惰层) 【yuánzǐdàn fǎnshècéng duòcéng】
regional system of accounting for and control of nuclear material (RSAC)	地区核材料衡算和控制系统 【dìqū hécáiliào héngsuàn hé kòngzhì xìtǒng】
Regulations of the People's Republic of China on Export Control of Dual-Use Nuclear Goods and the Related Technologies The chinese government promulgated the Regulations of the People's Republic of China on Export Control of Dual-use Nuclear Goods and the Related Technologies on June 10, 1998. The Regulations took effect as of the date of promulgation. They consist of 23 articles and the Annex named the Nuclear Dual-Use Items and Related	中华人民共和国核两用品及相关技术出口管制条例 【zhōnghuá rénmín gònghéguó hé liǎngyòngpǐn jí xiāngguān jìshù chūkǒu guǎnzhì tiáolì】 中国政府于 1998 年 6 月 10 日公布《中华人民共和国核两用品及相关技术出口管制条例》，条例从公布之日起生效。条例由 23 条正文和附件《核两用品及相关技术管制清单》组成。(源自：参考文献[1]，p415)

Technologies Export Control List. (From: Reference [1], p415) Note: this set of regulations was revised in 2007[73].	注：该条例在 2007 年被修订了[73]。
Regulations of the People's Republic of China on Nuclear Export Control The chinese government promulgated the Regulations of the People's Republic of China on Nuclear Export Control of on Sep.10, 1997, and declared that it took effect immediately. It has 22 articles. (From: Reference [1], p414) Note: this set of regulations was revised in 2006[74].	**中华人民共和国核出口管制条例【zhōnghuá rénmín gònghéguó hé chūkǒu guǎnzhì tiáolì】** 中国政府于 1997 年 9 月 10 日公布《中华人民共和国核出口管制条例》，并宣布立即生效。条例共 22 条。(源自：参考文献[1]，p414) 注：该条例在 2006 年被修订了[74]。
reliability of nuclear missiles	**核导弹可靠性【hédǎodàn kěkàoxìng】**
reliability of nuclear weapon Throughout the nuclear weapon's life-time, the capability to the achieve nuclear explosion within the designed performance under the defined normal environment. (Modified from: Reference [2], p221) Note 1: The probability of achieving the specified yield, at the target, across the Stockpile-To-Target Sequence of environments, throughout the weapon's lifetime, assuming proper inputs. In this definition, the specified yield is generally understood to mean within ten percent; the Stockpile-To-Target Sequence of environments is the range of conditions the warhead is expected to experience in its service life in storage, transit, or use, such as temperature extremes, radiation from any nuclear-armed missile defense interceptors, and acceleration; lifetime is the "original lifetime objective as	**核武器可靠性【héwǔqì kěkàoxìng】** 核武器在使用寿命期间，在规定的正常环境条件下，以设计性能指标实现核爆炸的能力。(改自：参考文献，[2] p221) 注 1：在核武器的整个设计寿命期间，经受从库存至打击目标的各种外部环境，在正确输入指令后，能在打击目标上实现指定威力的概率。在此定义中，"指定威力"通常被理解成与设计威力相差 10%以内的意思；"从库存至打击目标的环境"指核弹头在其服役期内的储存、转运和使用过程中会经历的外部环境，如极端温度、核导弹防御拦截器的辐射、过载；"寿命"指在设计时指定的初始寿命目标；"正确

specified at the time of design"; and proper inputs are arming, fuzing, and firing signals. (From: Reference[10], p8.) Note 2: In this definition from Sandia National Laboratories, "weapon" has the meaning of "warhead"; if "weapon" had the meaning of "weapon system" including the missile or aircraft, the reliability would be much lower.	输入"指引爆控制信号。(源自：参考文献[10]，p8) 注 2：圣地亚国家实验室的定义中，"武器"有"核弹头"的意思；如果"武器"有包含导弹或飞行器的"武器系统"的意思，那么可靠性将更低。
reliability of stockpile nuclear weapon	库存核武器可靠性【kùcún héwǔqì kěkàoxìng】
remote sensing technology Technology for detecting objects and/or activities at a distance by means of sensors. (Modified from: Reference [19], p235)	遥感技术【yáogǎn jìshù】 用传感器远距离探测与条约有关的物项和(或)活动的技术。(改自：参考文献[19]，p235)
representative sample	代表性样品【dàibiǎoxìng yàngpǐn】
reprocessing	后处理【hòuchǔlǐ】
reprocessing plant	后处理厂【hòuchǔlǐ chǎng】
research reactor	研究堆【yánjiūduī】
response time of nuclear missiles The time elapsed from receiving launch orders to the launch of nuclear missiles. (From: Reference [2], p50)	核导弹反应时间【hédǎodàn fǎnyìng shíjiān】 核导弹从接到发射命令到导弹起飞所需的时间。(源自：参考文献[2]，p50)
responsive force The responsive force is intended to provide a capability to augment the operationally deployed force to meet potential contingencies. It retains the option for leadership to increase the number of operationally deployed forces in proportion to the severity of an evolving crisis. (Modified from: Reference [66])	响应力量【xiǎngyìng lìliàng】 意指在遭遇潜在的意外事故时能增加作战部署力量的能力。它使领导层能握有根据危机发展的程度而增加作战部署力量数量的选择权。 (改自：参考文献[66])
retained waste	存留废物【cúnliú fèiwù】

E-C

E-C

retargeting capability	重新瞄准能力 【chóngxīn miáozhǔn nénglì】
revised supplementary agreement relevant to safeguards	有关保障监督的修订补充协定 【yǒuguān bǎozhàng jiāndū de xiūdìng bǔchōng xiédìng】
revisit period	重访周期 【chóngfǎng zhōuqī】
revolution in military affairs (RMA) Fundamental reforms that thoroughly change the characteristics and patterns of military operations so as to greatly enhance operational effectiveness of the military through advanced technology and weapons systems combined with innovative military doctrines and organizational mechanisms. (Modified from: Reference [1], p47)	军事变革【jūnshì biàngé】 将先进的技术和武器系统，与创新的军事学说和组织体制结合在一起，使军事作战的特点和方式发生根本性的变化，军队的作战效能达到极大提高的根本性改革。(改自：参考文献[1]，p47)
rotor of a gas centrifuge	气体离心机转筒 【qìtǐ líxīnjī zhuàntǒng】
routine inspection	例行视察【lìxíng shìchá】
Safeguards Agreement	保障监督协定 【bǎozhàng jiāndū xiédìng】
safeguards conclusion	保障监督结论 【bǎozhàng jiāndū jiélùn】
safeguards criteria	保障监督标准 【bǎozhàng jiāndū biāozhǔn】
Safeguards of International Atomic Energy Agency IAEA safeguards are a set of activities by which the IAEA seeks to verify that a State is living up to its international undertakings not to use peaceful nuclear programs for nuclear weapons purposes. The safeguards system is based on assessment of the correctness and completeness of the	国际原子能机构保障监督制度 【guójì yuánzǐnéng jīgòu bǎozhàng jiāndū zhìdù】 IAEA 的保障监督制度是 IAEA 为核实某国家履行未将民用核计划转用于核武器目的的国际承诺的一整套行动。保障监督体系是基于某国就其核材料和相关核活动向 IAEA

State's declarations to the IAEA concerning nuclear material and nuclear-related activities. To date, 145 States have entered into such agreements with the IAEA, submitting nuclear materials, facilities and activities to the scrutiny of IAEA's safeguards inspectors. IAEA verification helps to provide assurance that such items are not diverted or misused in order to assemble nuclear weapons and that no items required to be declared under safeguards are undeclared. (From: Reference[51])	申报的准确性和完整性的评估。迄今为止，已有 145 个国家加入 IAEA 的保障监督协议，将核材料、核设施和核活动呈交 IAEA 保障监督视查员进行详细审查。IAEA 的核查有助于确认上述项目未转用或滥用于制造核武器，以及保障监督所要求申报的项目已全部申报。(源自：参考文献[51])
safeguards quality assurance In the context of IAEA safeguards, a management tool for ensuring a systematic approach to all of the activities affecting the quality of the safeguards implementation. (From: Reference [4], 3.36)	保障监督的质量保证 【bǎozhàng jiāndū de zhìliàng bǎozhèng】 在国际原子能机构保障监督体系下，确保对所有会影响保障监督实施质量的活动进行系统化监控的一种管理手段。(源自：参考文献[4]，3.36)
safety problems of atmospheric nuclear test	大气层核试验的安全问题 【dàqìcéng héshìyàn de ānquán wèntí】
safety problems of under-ground nuclear test	地下核试验的安全问题 【dìxià héshìyàn de ānquán wèntí】
safing device of nuclear weapon Refer to "**permissive action link (PAL)**"	核武器保险装置 【héwǔqì bǎoxiǎn zhuāngzhì】 参见"密码锁(亦称启动连接装置)"
sample	样品【yàngpǐn】
sample size	样品量【yàngpǐnliàng】
sampling technology of atmospheric nuclear explosion	大气层核爆炸取样技术 【dàqìcéng hébàozhà qǔyàng jìshù】
sampling technology of underground nuclear explosion	地下核爆炸取样技术 【dìxià hébàozhà qǔyàng jìshù】
scaled depth of burst	比例爆深【bǐlì bàoshēn】

E I C

scaled height of burst	比例爆高【bǐlì bàogāo】
scrap	切削(碎)料【qiēxuē suì liào】
scrap recovery plant	切削(碎)料回收厂 【qiēxuē suì liào huíshōuchǎng】
seal Anything that tightly or completely closes or secures a thing. A seal with special markers is usually applied to those inspected equipments or components in order to prevent weapons and related components from being transferred and modified. A seal must be tamper-proof and counterfeit-proof and it must be unique and hard to duplicate with high confidence. It also should guarantee that inspected equipments or components remain unaffected or unchanged and that sensitive information related to the inspected facilities would not be revealed. Seals currently in application include fiber seal, welding seal, electric seal and ultrasonic seal etc. (From: Reference [1], p496) Note: An active seal requires electrical power, while a passive seal works without a power supply.	封记【fēngjì】 用以紧紧地或完全地封闭或保护某物，俗称封条或封签。利用做特殊标记的方法在被核查设备或部件加封条，以防止武器及武器部件被转移和改动的措施。封记必须具有防止篡改和防伪造的特性，具有唯一性，不能复制，有很强的置信度，同时又要保证被核查设备或部件不受影响或不被改变，不揭示被核查设施的敏感信息。应用中的封记有光纤封记、焊缝封记、电子封记和超声封记等。(源自：参考文献[1]，p496) 注：有源封记工作时需要电源，但无源封记不需要电源。
second-generation nuclear weapon	第二代核武器【dì'èrdài héwǔqì】
seismic monitoring	地震监测【dìzhèn jiāncè】
seismic monitoring system	地震监测系统【dìzhèn jiāncè xìtǒng】
self-defensive nuclear counterattack A nuclear counterattack launched after absorbing an opponent's first nuclear attack. (Modified from: Reference [34])	自卫核反击【zìwèi héfǎnjī】 在遭受第一次核打击后进行核反击。(改自：参考文献[34])
self-defensive nuclear strategy Term used officially by China to	自卫防御核战略 【zìwèi fángyù hézhànlüè】

describe its nuclear strategy. The strategy takes as its fundamental goal deterring other countries from using or threatening to use nuclear weapons against China. It includes an official commitment to a policy of no first use of nuclear weapons at any time and under any circumstances. It unconditionally undertakes not to use or threaten to use nuclear weapons against non-nuclear-weapon states or nuclear-weapon-free zones, and stands for the comprehensive prohibition and complete elimination of nuclear weapons. The strategy upholds the principles of counterattack in self-defense and limited development of nuclear weapons, and aims at building a lean and effective nuclear force capable of meeting national security needs. It endeavors to ensure the security and reliability of its nuclear weapons and maintains a credible nuclear deterrent force. (Modified from: Reference [34])	中国官方描述其核战略所用的术语。该战略的根本目标是遏制他国对中国使用或威胁使用核武器。该战略正式承诺在任何时候、任何情况下都不首先使用核武器的政策，无条件地承诺不对无核国家和无核地区使用或威胁使用核武器，主张全面禁止和彻底销毁核武器。该战略坚持自卫反击和有限发展的原则，着眼于建设一支满足国家安全需要的精干有效的核力量，确保核武器的安全性、可靠性，保持核力量的战略威慑作用。(改自：参考文献[34])
self-destruct device of nuclear weapon	核武器自毁装置【héwǔqì zìhuǐ zhuāngzhì】
self-sustaining thermonuclear burn	自持热核燃烧【zìchí rèhé ránshāo】
separation efficiency of a countercurrent gas centrifuge	逆流气体离心机的分离效率【nìliú qìtǐ líxīnjī de fēnlí xiàolǜ】
separation stage	分离级【fēnlíjí】
separative element	分离单元【fēnlí dānyuán】
separative power A unit for measuring separative work per unit time provided by a separating unit or a separating cascade. (Modified from: Reference [2], p125)	分离功率【fēnlí gōnglǜ】 一个分离单元或一个分离级联在单位时间所能提供的分离功。(改自：参考文献[2]，p125)

separative work The required work to enrich uranium to a certain level of U-235 concentration. It is described in terms of kg Separative Work Unit (kgSWU) or ton Separative Work Unit (tSWU). (From：Reference [26], p213)	分离功【fēnlígōng】 把一定量的铀浓缩到一定的铀-235丰度所需要投入的工作量，表达为千克分离功单位(kgSWU)或吨分离功单位(tSWU)。 (源自：参考文献[26]，p213)
separative work unit	分离功单位【fēnlígōng dānwèi】
service safety	勤务保险【qínwù bǎoxiǎn】
shaft nuclear test	竖井地下核试验 【shùjǐng dìxià héshìyàn】
shipper/receiver difference (SRD)	发方/收方差额 【fāfāng shōufāng chā'é】
shock wave load	冲击载荷【chōngjī zàihè】
shock wave weapon	冲击波弹【chōngjībō dàn】
short-notice inspection An inspection performed at a facility or a location outside facilities for which less advance notice is provided by the IAEA to the State than that provided for under paragraph 83 of [IAEA INFIRCIR 153]. (From: Reference [4], 11.7)	临时通知视察【línshí tōngzhī shìchá】 IAEA 对一个国家的一处设施或设施外的一处场地进行视察时，提前通报时间比 INFIRCIR/153 协议的第 83 段规定的通报时间短的视察。 (源自：参考文献[4]，11.7)
significant quantity (SQ) The approximate amount of nuclear material for which the possibility of manufacturing a nuclear explosive device cannot be excluded. (From: Reference [4], 3.14)	重要量【zhòngyàoliàng】 不能排除制造一枚核爆炸装置可能性的核材料的大致数量。(源自：参考文献[4]，3.14)
silo	地下发射井【dìxià fāshèjǐng】
silo cold launch	地下井冷发射【dìxiàjǐng lěngfāshè】
silo hot launch	地下井热发射【dìxiàjǐng rèfāshè】
simulation of nuclear explosion	核爆炸模拟【hébàozhà mónǐ】

simulation of nuclear explosion effects Using various simulating measures to research the destructive mechanisms and protective measures against the effects of a nuclear explosion. (Modified from: Reference [3], p377)	**核爆炸效应模拟** 【hébàozhà xiàoyìng mónǐ】 利用各种模拟手段研究核爆炸破坏机理以及对核爆炸效应的保护措施。(改自：参考文献[3]，p377)
simultaneous inspections Inspections performed by IAEA inspectors simultaneously or within a short period of time at two or more facilities in a State in order to detect possible diversions arranged in collusion between facilities by, for example, the temporary transfer ("borrowing") of nuclear material between facilities so that the same material would be verified twice by the IAEA, once in each of the two facilities inspected. (From: Reference [4], 11.11)	**同时视察**【tóngshí shìchá】 IAEA 视察员同时或在短时间内对一个国家的两处或多处设施进行视察，以发现设施之间可能进行的串通行为，例如设施之间相互临时转移(借用)核材料，从而使同一份核材料被 IAEA 核查两次，即在两个被视察的设施中各被核查一次。(源自：参考文献[4]，11.11)
single-cycle process	**单循环流程**【dānxúnhuán liúchéng】
slow neutrons	**慢中子**【màn zhōngzǐ】
small quantities protocol (SQP)	**小数量议定书** 【xiǎoshùliàng yìdìngshū】
source data	**原始数据**【yuánshǐ shùjù】
source material Uranium containing the mixture of isotopes occurring in nature; uranium depleted in the isotope 235; thorium; any of the foregoing in the form of metal, alloy, chemical compound, or concentrate; any other material containing one or more of the foregoing in such concentration as the IAEA Board of Governors shall from time to time determine; and such other material as the Board of Governors shall from	**源材料**【yuáncáiliào】 含有天然形成的同位素混合体的铀；铀-235 被贫化的铀；钍；金属、合金、化合物或浓缩物状态的上述任何材料；任何含有一种或多种上述的物质并达到 IAEA 理事会随时确定的浓度的材料；以及理事会可随时确定的此类其他材料。根据[INFIRCIR/153]保障协定的 112 段：

E I C

time to time determine. According to paragraph 112 of [IAEA INFCIRC/153], "the term source material shall not be interpreted as applying to ore or ore residue." (From: Reference [4], 4.4)	"源材料这一名词不适用于矿石或矿渣。"(源自：参考文献[4]，4.4)
South Pacific Nuclear Free Zone Treaty (Treaty of Rarotonga)	**南太平洋无核区条约(拉罗汤加岛条约)** 【nántàipíngyáng wúhéqū tiáoyuē lāluótāngjiādǎo tiáoyuē】
spare warhead	**备用弹头**【bèiyòng dàntóu】
special fissionable material Plutonium-239; uranium-233; uranium enriched in the isotopes 235 or 233; any material containing one or more of the foregoing; and such other fissionable material as the IAEA Board of Governors shall from time to time determine; but the term "special fissionable material" does not include source material. (From: Reference [4], 4.5)	**特种可裂变材料** 【tèzhǒng kělièbiàn cáiliào】 钚-239；铀-233；浓缩了同位素铀-235 或铀-233 的铀；任何含上述一种或多种物质的材料；以及 IAEA 理事会随时确定的其他可裂变材料；但"特种可裂变材料"不包括源材料。(源自：参考文献[4]，4.5)
special inspection An inspection is deemed to be special: when it either is additional to the routine inspection effort provided for in paragraphs 78–82 of [IAEA INFCIRC/153], or involves access to information or locations in addition to the access specified in paragraph 76 of [IAEA INFCIRC/153] for ad hoc and routine inspections, or both. (From: Reference [4], 11.13; [15])	**专门视察**【zhuānmén shìchá】 一种在以下情况下进行的、被认为是很特殊的视察：在 INFIRCIR/153 协议中第 78-82 段规定的常规视察要求之外进行的视察；或者是想通过获取或进入除 INFIRCIR/153 协议中第 76 段特别指明的可以进入的信息或场地之外的信息或场地进行的特别的和常规的视察；或者以上两种情况都包括的视察。(源自：参考文献[4] 11.13；[15])
Special Session of the General Assembly Devoted to Disarmament	**联大裁军特别会议** 【liándà cáijūn tèbié huìyì】

specified equipment	规定的设备【guīdìng de shèbèi】
spectral resolution	谱分辨率【pǔ fēnbiànlǜ】
spent fuel	乏燃料【fáránliào】
Spent Fuel Management Safety and Radioactive Waste Management Safety Joint Convention	乏燃料管理安全和放射性废物管理安全联合公约【fáránliào guǎnlǐ ānquán hé fàngshè xìng fèiwù guǎnlǐ ānquán liánhé gōngyuē】
spent fuel storage	乏燃料贮存【fáránliào zhùcún】
spontaneous fission	自发裂变【zìfā lièbiàn】
stage separation efficiency of gaseous diffusion process	气体扩散分离级的分离效率【qìtǐ kuòsàn fēnlíjí de fēnlí xiàolǜ】
standard event screening criteria	标准事件筛选判据【biāozhǔn shìjiàn shāixuǎn pànjù】
standby facility	停产的设施【tíngchǎn de shèshī】
starting point of IAEA safe-guards	国际原子能机构保障监督的起点【guójì yuánzǐnéng jīgòu bǎozhàng jiāndū de qǐdiǎn】
state-level safeguards approach A safeguards approach developed for a specific State, encompassing all nuclear material, nuclear installations and nuclear fuel cycle related activities in that State. (From: Reference [4], 3.4)	国家级保障监督方案【guójiājí bǎozhàng jiāndū fāng'àn】 为具体国家制定的保障监督方案，方案涵盖该国所有与核材料、核设施以及与核燃料循环相关的活动。(源自：参考文献[4]，3.4)
state system of accounting for and control of nuclear material (SSAC)	国家核材料衡算和控制系统【guójiā hécáiliào héngsuàn hé kòngzhì xìtǒng】
statement	声明【shēngmíng】
statute	规约【guīyuē】
Statute of the International Atomic Energy Agency	国际原子能机构规约【guójì yuánzǐnéng jīgòu guīyuē】
Stockpile Stewardship and Management Program	核武库维护与管理计划【héwǔkù wéihù yǔ guǎnlǐ jìhuà】

storage and custody of nuclear weapon	核武器贮存与保管【héwǔqì zhùcún yǔ bǎoguǎn】
storage environment of nuclear weapon	核武器贮存环境【héwǔqì zhùcún huánjìng】
storage facility	贮存设施【zhùcún shèshī】
storage life of nuclear weapon	核武器贮存期【héwǔqì zhùcúnqī】
strategic defense 1 The defense against an offensive enemy in the overall situation of war. It is one of the basic types of strategic operations and usually becomes a stage in the course of war. The aim of strategic defense is to prevent and frustrate the enemy's strategic offense, preserve and save one's own strength, wear down and wipe out the enemy, change the battle situation and relative strength, and create conditions for shifting to strategic offense. (From: Reference [18], p219) 2 The capability to defeat an enemy's use of its strategic military assets, primarily long-range nuclear delivery systems. (Modified from: Reference [71])	战略防御【zhànlüè fángyù】 1 战争全局上对进攻之敌的防御。它是战争中战略行动的基本类型之一，往往成为战争进程的一个阶段。战略防御的目的是阻止和挫败敌人的战略进攻，保存和积蓄自己的力量，消耗和消灭敌人，改变战场形势和力量对比，为转入战略进攻创造条件。(源自：参考文献[18]，p219) 2 挫伤敌人使用战略军事设施(主要是远程核运载系统)的能力。(改自：参考文献[71])
strategic defense initiative (SDI) The plan for a space-based ballistic missile defense system announced by U.S. president Ronald Reagan on March 23, 1983, aimed at defending against a mass attack of strategic nuclear missiles from the Soviet Union. It is also commonly called "Star Wars". (Modified from: Reference [1], p274；[17])	战略防御倡议【zhànlüè fángyù chàngyì】 罗纳德·里根总统在 1983 年 3 月 23 日声明的《战略防御倡议》指为拦截苏联射向美国的大规模战略导弹力量而建立的天基弹道导弹防御系统研制计划，俗称“星球大战”计划。(改自：参考文献[1]，p274；[17])
strategic missile	战略导弹【zhànlüè dǎodàn】
strategic nuclear weapon 1 Nuclear weapons that are used to	战略核武器【zhànlüè héwǔqì】 1 用于打击战略目标，执行战略任

strike strategic targets for strategic missions. (Modified from: Reference [3], p1105) 2 Strategic nuclear weapons are designed to engage objects in geographically remote strategic regions (over 5 500 km) to accomplish strategic missions. In exceptional situations, strategic nuclear weapons may be used to accomplish campaign missions. Strategic nuclear weapons are in service with the strategic nuclear forces. (From: Reference [5], p24) Note: Strategic refers to missions designed to have a long-term rather than immediate effect on the enemy and its military forces. (Modified from: Reference [9], p516-517) Refer to "**tactical nuclear weapon**"	务的核武器。(改自：参考文献[3],p1105) 2 战略核武器是指能打击远距离地域的战略目标(超过 5 500 公里)完成战略任务的武器。特殊情况下战略核武器可用于完成战役任务。战略核武器服役于战略核部队。(源自：参考文献[5]，p24) 注：战略担负对敌方及其军事力量产生长期的而非短期影响的使命。(改自：参考文献[9]，p516-517) 参见"战术核武器"
strategic point	战略要点【zhànlüè yàodiǎn】
strategic stability	战略稳定性【zhànlüè wěndìngxìng】
strategy of flexible response	灵活反应战略 【línghuó fǎnyìng zhànlüè】
strategy of going beyond containment	超越遏制战略 【chāoyuè èzhì zhànlüè】
strategy of massive retaliation	大规模报复战略 【dàguīmó bàofù zhànlüè】
strategy of mutual assured destruction (MAD)	相互确保摧毁战略 【xiānghù quèbǎocuīhuǐ zhànlüè】
strategy of realistic deterrence	现实威慑战略 【xiànshí wēishè zhànlüè】
subcritical assembly	次临界装置【cìlínjiè zhuāngzhì】
subcritical experiment Hydrodynamic detonation experiment in which the fission system remains subcritical, the material used would not	次临界实验【cìlínjiè shíyàn】 实验中裂变系统处于次临界状态的爆轰流体动力学实验，裂变材料的

exceed the amount that may produce a self-sustaining chain reaction. (Modified from: Reference [1], p214)	用量以不会发生自持链式裂变核反应为限。(改自:参考文献[1]，p214)
subcritical gas centrifuge	亚临界气体离心机【yàlínjiè qìtǐ líxīnjī】
subcritical safety simulation experiment system	次临界安全模拟实验系统【cìlínjiè ānquán mónǐ shíyàn xìtǒng】
subcriticality	次临界度【cìlínjiè dù】
submarine-launched ballistic missile	潜射弹道导弹【qiánshè dàndàodǎodàn】
supercritical gas centrifuge	超临界气体离心机【chāolínjiè qìtǐ líxīnjī】
surveillance of nuclear material	核材料监视【hécáiliào jiānshì】
survivability of nuclear weapon Capability for nuclear weapons on active service to remain intact after another country launches a first nuclear strike. (From: Reference [2], p222)	核武器生存能力【héwǔqì shēngcún nénglì】 一方的现役核武器在对方进行第一次核打击后保持完好的能力。(源自：参考文献[2]，p222)
suspect-site inspection	可疑场地视察【kěyí chǎngdì shìchá】
suspension of IAEA safeguards	国际原子能机构保障监督的中止【guójì yuánzǐnéng jīgòu bǎozhàng jiāndū de zhōngzhǐ】
suspension protocol	暂停实施议定书【zàntíng shíshī yìdìngshū】
swipe samples of nuclear material	核材料擦拭样品【hécáiliào cāshì yàngpǐn】
swipe sampling The collection of environmental samples by swiping a surface with a piece of ultraclean medium (such as cloth) to remove from the surface traces of the materials present. (From: Reference [4], 9.4)	擦拭取样【cāshì qǔyàng】 一种环境样品的收集方法，它通过用一块超洁净介质(例如布)擦拭物体表面以获取物体表面残留的材料痕迹。(源自：参考文献[4]，9.4)
synthetic aperture radar (SAR)	合成孔径雷达【héchéng kǒngjìng léidá】

systematic sampling The process of selecting samples in a repeated pattern, such as every 11th item or at fixed time intervals, from a continuing process. (From: Reference [4], 7.9)	**系统取样【xìtǒng qǔyàng】** 在一个连续的过程中以重复的方式进行取样，如每隔 10 个物项取样或每隔一定的时间间隔取样。(源自：参考文献[4]，7.9)
system-generated electromagnetic pulse	**系统电磁脉冲【xìtǒng diàncí màichōng】**
tactical missile	**战术导弹【zhànshù dǎodàn】**
tactical nuclear weapon 1 Nuclear weapons used to attack in-depth key targets at the campaign and tactical level. (Modified from: Reference [3], p1107)	**战术核武器【zhànshù héwǔqì】** 1 用于打击战役、战术纵深内重要目标的核武器。(改自：参考文献[3]，p1107)
2 Nuclear weapons, such as artillery shells, bombs, and short-range missiles, for use in battlefield operations. (Modified from: Reference [8])	2 用于战场作战的核武器，诸如核炮弹、核炸弹和短程核导弹等。(改自：参考文献[8])
3 Tactical nuclear weapons are designed to engage objects in the tactical depth of enemy deployment (up to 300 km) to accomplish a tactical mission. Under certain conditions, tactical nuclear weapons may be involved in operational and strategic missions. A strategic bomb can be used for tactical purposes. (Modified from: Reference [5], p24)	3 战术核武器是指能打击敌方部署的战术纵深目标(最远 300 公里)完成战术任务的武器。在某些情况下，战术核武器可用于作战和战略任务，战略核炸弹也可用于战术目的。(改自：参考文献[5]，p24)
Notes 1: Activities at a tactical level focus on the ordered arrangement and maneuver of combat elements in relation to each other and to the enemy to achieve combat objectives. (Modified from: Reference [9], p532)	注 1：战术层面的活动是为完成战斗目的而关注涉及己方和敌方的作战要素的部署和调遣。(改自：参考文献[9]，p532)
Note 2: A campaign is a series of combat operations carried out by	注 2：战役是指军团为达成战争的局部目的或全局性目的，在统一指

E I C

corps-level military forces under uniformed command to achieve partial or overall objectives. (From: Reference [33], p9) Refer to "**strategic nuclear weapon**"	挥下进行的由一系列战斗组成的作战行动。(源自：参考文献[33]，p9) 参见"**战略核武器**"
tag A unique identifier set up for facilitating verification of items restricted by arms control treaties. A tag must have intrinsic characteristic which make it difficult to be duplicated, transferred, tampered or detected. A tag should also be stable, credible and inexpensive. (From: Reference [1], p496) Note: An active tag requires electrical power, while a passive tag works without a power supply.	**标签【biāoqiān】** 在军备控制条约的限制对象上，为便于核查而设置的某种独特标志。标签必须具有固有的特征，不能复制、转移、篡改或探测，同时要稳定、可靠、便宜。(源自：参考文献[1]，p496) 注：有源标签工作时需要电源，但无源标签不需要电源。
tailored deterrence Flexible deterrence capabilities and operational doctrines specifically designed according to the specific psychological, political, ideological, and economic characteristics of the targeted actor. (From: Reference[21], p49-51)	**针对性威慑【zhēnduìxìng wēishè】** 根据目标国具体的心理、政治、意识形态，及经济状况而特别制订的灵活的威摄能力与实战原则。(源自：参考文献[21]，p49-51)
tailored effects nuclear weapon	**特殊效应核武器【tèshū xiàoyìng héwǔqì】**
tamper resistance	**抗干扰【kàng gānrǎo】**
tampering	**干扰【gānrǎo】**
target-changing capability	**变换打击目标能力【biànhuàn dǎjī mùbiāo nénglì】**
target of nuclear strike	**核打击目标【hédǎjī mùbiāo】**
target positioning	**目标定位【mùbiāo dìngwèi】**
technical characteristics exhibition and inspection	**技术特性展示和视察【jìshù tèxìng zhǎnshì hé shìchá】**

technologies for on-site inspection of nuclear explosion	核爆炸现场视察技术 【hébàozhà xiànchǎng shìchá jìshù】
telemetry data packet encryption	遥测数据打包和加密 【yáocè shùjù dǎbāo hé jiāmì】
telemetry signal for missiles	导弹遥测信号【dǎodàn yáocè xìnhào】
telemetry system for nuclear weapon	核武器遥测系统 【héwǔqì yáocè xìtǒng】
template approach The template approach to identify treaty-limited objects works by measuring certain characteristics of an object and comparing them with the same set of measurements taken from a reference object (e.g., an authentic weapon of a particular type): the template. (From: Reference [11], p99)	模板法【móbǎnfǎ】 模板法是通过测量物体的某些特征，并与从某个参照物(如经认证的一件特定类型的武器)测得的同样一组特征(即模板)相比较。如果这两组数据测量相符，就可以判定该物体就是这种类型的武器。(源自：参考文献[11]，p99)
temporal resolution	时间分辨率 【shíjiān fēnbiànlǜ】
Ten Principles of the Bandung Conference	万隆会议十项原则 【wànlóng huìyì shíxiàng yuánzé】
Ten-Nation Committee on Disarmament (TNCD)	十国裁军委员会 【shíguó cáijūn wěiyuánhuì】
termination of IAEA safeguards	国际原子能机构保障监督的终止 【guójì yuánzǐnéng jīgòu bǎozhàng jiāndū de zhōngzhǐ】
theater nuclear weapon	战区核武器【zhànqū héwǔqì】
theoretical maximum separative power of a gas centrifuge	气体离心机的最大理论分离功率 【qìtǐ líxīnjī de zuìdà lǐlùn fēnlí gōnglǜ】
theory of cascade	级联理论【jílián lǐlùn】
theory of escalation	逐步升级论【zhúbù shēngjílùn】
theory of low intensity conflict	低强度冲突理论 【dīqiángdù chōngtū lǐlùn】

E-C

theory of peaceful settlement	和平解决理论【hépíng jiějué lǐlùn】
theory of victory decided by nuclear weapons	核武器制胜论【héwǔqì zhìshènglùn】
thermal neutrons	热中子【rèzhōngzǐ】
thermal radiation of nuclear explosion	核爆炸光(热)辐射 【hébàozhà guāngrèfúshè】
thermonuclear ignition	热核点火【rèhé diǎnhuǒ】
thermonuclear weapon	热核武器【rèhéwǔqì】
third-generation nuclear weapon	第三代核武器【dìsāndài héwǔqì】
THOREX (thorium extraction) process	梭雷克斯流程【suōléikèsī liúchéng】 (钍萃取流程)
thorium-uranium nuclear fuel cycle	钍-铀核燃料循环 【tǔ yóu héránliào xúnhuán】
Three Principles on Nuclear Export Control of China China's three principles of nuclear exports: guarantee for peaceful purposes only; acceptance of IAEA safeguards; and no retransfer to any third party without prior approval of the Chinese side. (From: Reference [1], p414)	中国核出口三项原则 【zhōngguó héchūkǒu sānxiàng yuánzé】 中国核出口三项原则：第一，只用于和平目的；第二，接受国际原子能机构的保障和监督；第三，未经中国同意，接受国不得转让给第三国。(源自：参考文献[1]，p414)
throw weight of nuclear missile	核导弹投掷重量 【hédǎodàn tóuzhì zhòngliàng】
TNT equivalent	梯恩梯当量【tī'ēntī dāngliàng】
transfer guideline	转让准则【zhuǎnràng zhǔnzé】
transient radiation effects on electronics	电子系统的瞬态辐射效应 【diànzǐ xìtǒng de shùntài fúshè xiàoyìng】
transmutation	嬗变【shànbiàn】
transparency Openness of information. In the verification field it may refer to openness about	透明度【tòumíngdù】 信息公开。在核查领域可指国家军事活动和可能带有军事意味的和平

a state's military activities and about any peaceful activities that may have military implications (such as dual-use technology). (From: Reference [54])	活动(如军民两用技术)的公开。(源自：参考文献[54])
treatment of radioactive solid waste	放射性固体废物处理【fàngshèxìng gùtǐ fèiwù chǔlǐ】
Treaty Banning Nuclear Weapon Tests in the Atmosphere, in Outer Space and Under Water (PTBT)	禁止在大气层、外层空间和水下进行核武器试验条约【jìnzhǐ zài dàqìcéng wàicéng kōngjiān hé shuǐxià jìnxíng héwǔqì shìyàn tiáoyuē】
Treaty Between the United States of America and the Russian Federation on Further Reduction and Limitation of Strategic Offensive Arms (START II)	美俄关于进一步削减和限制进攻性战略武器条约【měi é guānyú jìnyībù xuējiǎn hé xiànzhì jìngōngxìng zhànlüè wǔqì tiáoyuē】
Treaty Between the United States of America and the Russian Federation on Strategic Offensive Reductions (Moscow/SORT)	美俄削减进攻性战略武器条约(莫斯科条约)【měi é xuējiǎn jìngōngxìng zhànlüè wǔqì tiáoyuē mòsīkē tiáoyuē】
Treaty Between the United States of America and the Union of Soviet Socialist Republics on the Elimination of Their Intermediate-Range and Shorter-Range Missiles (INF Treaty)	美苏关于消除两国中程及中短程导弹条约(中导条约)【měi sū guānyú xiāochú liǎngguó zhōngchéng jí zhōngduǎnchéng dǎodàn tiáoyuē zhōngdǎo tiáoyuē】
Treaty Between the United States of America and the Union of Soviet Socialist Republics on the Limitation of Anti-ballistic Missile Systems (ABM Treaty)	美苏关于限制反弹道导弹系统条约(反导条约)【měi sū guānyú xiànzhì fǎn dàndàodǎodàn xìtǒng tiáoyuē fǎndǎo tiáoyuē】
Treaty Between the United States of America and the Union of Soviet Socialist Republics on the Limitation of Strategic Offensive Arms (SALT II Treaty)	美苏限制进攻性战略武器条约【měi sū xiànzhì jìngōngxìng zhànlüè wǔqì tiáoyuē】

Treaty Between the United States of America and the Union of Soviet Socialist Republics on the Limitation of Underground Nuclear Weapon Tests (TTBT)	美苏限制地下核武器试验条约(限当量条约) 【měi sū xiànzhì dìxià héwǔqì shìyàn tiáoyuē xiàndāngliàng tiáoyuē】
Treaty Between the United States of America and the Union of Soviet Socialist Republics on the Reduction and Limitation of Offensive Strategic Arms (START I)	美苏关于削减和限制进攻性战略武器条约 【měi sū guānyú xuējiǎn hé xiànzhì jìngōngxìng zhànlüèwǔqì tiáoyuē】
Treaty Between the United States of America and the Union of Soviet Socialist Republics on Underground Nuclear Explosion for Peaceful Purposes (PNE)	美苏和平利用地下核爆炸条约 【měi sū hépíng lìyòng dìxià hébàozhà tiáoyuē】
Treaty for the Prohibition of Nuclear Weapons in Latin America and the Caribbean (Treaty of Tlatelolco)	拉丁美洲和加勒比海禁止核武器条约 【lādīngměizhōu hé jiālèbǐhǎi jìnzhǐ héwǔqì tiáoyuē】
Treaty on the Non-Proliferation of Nuclear Weapons (NPT)	不扩散核武器条约 【bùkuòsàn héwǔqì tiáoyuē】
Treaty on the Southeast Asia Nuclear Weapon-Free Zone (Treaty of Bangkok)	东南亚无核武器区条约(曼谷条约) 【dōngnányà wúhéwǔqìqū tiáoyuē màngǔ tiáoyuē】
triad strategic nuclear force Refer to **"old nuclear triad"**	三位一体战略核力量 【sānwèiyītǐ zhànlüè hélìliàng】 参见"旧核三位一体"
trigger list The NSG prescribes that items on the list exported to non-nuclear-weapon states should trigger the IAEA safe-guards. (From: Reference [1], p407)	触发清单【chùfā qīngdān】 核供应国集团规定，向无核武器国家出口"清单"上的项目，要"触发"国际原子能机构的保障监督。 (源自：参考文献[1]，p407)
tri-phase bomb A type of hydrogen bomb whose energy release process consists of three	三相弹【sānxiàngdàn】 放能过程经历由裂变到聚变再到裂

phases: fission, fusion, and then fission. The final fission phase is achieved by the use of natural uranium, depleted uranium, or enriched uranium in proximity to the thermonuclear fuel. Most strategic nuclear weapons in the world belong to this type. (Modified from: Reference [3], p802)	变三个阶段的一种氢弹，其最后的裂变阶段由临近于热核燃料的天然铀、贫铀或浓缩铀来完成。世界上大多数战略核武器都属于这种类型。(改自：参考文献[3]，p802)
tritium	氚【chuān】
tritium production reactor	产氚堆【chǎn chuān duī】
tunnel nuclear test	平洞地下核试验【píngdòng dìxià héshìyàn】
two cycle process	双循环流程【shuāngxúnhuán liúchéng】
type (environment) of nuclear explosion Nuclear weapons or nuclear explosive devices can be exploded in different media or at different heights/depths, in the atmosphere, in space, underwater and underground. (Modified from: Reference [1], p191)	核爆炸方式(环境)【hébàozhà fāngshì huánjìng】核武器或核爆炸装置在不同介质、不同高度或深度的爆炸，包括大气层核爆炸、高空核爆炸、水下核爆炸和地下核爆炸等。(改自：参考文献[1]，p191)
UN General Assembly	联合国大会【liánhéguó dàhuì】
UN resolution concerning the definition of aggression	联合国关于侵略定义的决议【liánhéguó guānyú qīnlüè dìngyì de juéyì】
unannounced inspection	不通知视察【bùtōngzhī shìchá】
undeclared facility or location outside facilities (LOF)	未申报设施或设施外场所【wèi shēnbào shèshī huò shèshīwài chǎngsuǒ】
underground nuclear test	地下核试验【dìxià héshìyàn】
unified uranium	合计铀【héjì yóu】
United Nations Advisory Board on Disarmament Affairs	联合国裁军事务咨询委员会【liánhéguó cáijūn shìwù zīxún wěiyuánhuì】

United Nations Charter	联合国宪章【liánhéguó xiànzhāng】
United Nations Commission for Conventional Armaments	联合国常规军备委员会【liánhéguó chángguī jūnbèi wěiyuánhuì】
United Nations Disarmament Commission (UNDC)	联合国裁军审议委员会【liánhéguó cáijūn shěnyì wěiyuánhuì】
United Nations Institute for Disarmament Research (UNIDIR)	联合国裁军研究所【liánhéguó cáijūn yánjiūsuǒ】
United Nations Office (Department) for Disarmament Affairs	联合国裁军事务部【liánhéguó cáijūn shìwùbù】
United Nations Register of Conventional Weapons	联合国常规武器转让登记册【liánhéguó chángguī wǔqì zhuǎnràng dēngjìcè】
uranium	铀【yóu】
uranium alloy	铀合金【yóu héjīn】
uranium chemical concentrate	铀化学浓缩物【yóu huàxué nóngsuōwù】
uranium decontamination cycle	铀净化循环【yóu jìnghuà xúnhuán】
uranium dioxide	二氧化铀【èryǎnghuàyóu】
uranium hexafluoride	六氟化铀【liùfúhuàyóu】
uranium hexafluoride hydrolysis	六氟化铀水解【liùfúhuàyóu shuǐjiě】
uranium isotope separation	铀同位素分离【yóu tóngwèisù fēnlí】
uranium mine and ore processing	铀矿开采和水冶【yóukuàng kāicǎi hé shuǐyě】
uranium purification plant	铀纯化厂【yóu chúnhuàchǎng】
uranium recycling A process of reusing the uranium extracted from spent fuel in nuclear reactors. (From: Reference [2], p457)	铀再循环【yóu zàixúnhuán】 将从乏燃料中回收得到的铀在反应堆内再循环使用的过程。(源自：参考文献[2]，p457)

uranium spectrum	铀光谱【yóu guāngpǔ】
uranium-233	铀-233【yóu 233】
uranium-plutonium cycle	铀钚循环【yóu bù xúnhuán】
uranium-plutonium mixed dioxide	铀钚混合氧化物 【yóu bù hùnhé yǎnghuàwù】
uranium-plutonium partition cycle	铀钚分离循环 【yóu bù fēnlí xúnhuán】
U.S. Nuclear Non-Proliferation Act of 1978 The Nuclear Non-Proliferation Act declares it United States policy: (1) to pursue the establishment of international controls of nuclear equipment, material, and technology, (2) to enhance the reliability of the United States as a supplier of nuclear reactors and fuels, (3) to encourage ratification of the Treaty on the Non-Proliferation of Nuclear Weapons, and (4) to aid other nations in identification and adaptation of appropriate energy production technology. (Modified from: Reference [35])	美国 1978 年核不扩散法 【měiguó 1978 nián hébùkuòsàn fǎ】 核不扩散法声明了美国的政策：(1)寻求建立核设备、核材料和核技术的国际控制；(2)提高美国作为核反应堆和核燃料供应国的可靠性；(3)鼓励批准《不扩散核武器条约》；(4)帮助其他国家核实和调整适当的能源生产技术。(改自：参考文献[35])
value function	价值函数【jiàzhí hánshù】
variable frequency power for special purpose of a centrifuge	离心机专用变频电源 【líxīnjī zhuānyòng biànpín diànyuán】
variance σ^2	方差 σ^2【fāngchā σ^2】
verification In the arms control field, it refers to the process of establishing whether state parties are complying with the provision of an agreement. It entails monitoring the activities of the parties relevant to their treaty commitments, analysing the information collected from monitoring, and determining whether the parties are complying with their agreement obligations. (Modified from: Reference [19], p237)	核查【héchá】 在军控中是指确认缔约国是否遵守协议条款的过程。它必须监测各缔约国有关条约承诺的活动，分析从监测收集的信息，并确定各缔约国是否遵守其对条约承诺的义务。 (改自：参考文献[19]，p237)

verification and validation (V&V) Verification is the process of confirming that a computer code correctly implements the algorithms that were intended. Validation is the process of confirming that the predictions of a code adequately represent measured physical phenomena. (Modified from: Reference [63])	**验证与确认【yànzhèng yǔ quèrèn】** 验证：是一个确定过程，即验证计算程序正确地求解了数学方程的过程。 确认：也是一个确定过程，即确认计算程序的计算结果恰当地描述了相关物理现象的过程。(改自：参考文献[63])
verification of the fissile material production cutoff	**禁止生产易裂变材料核查【jìnzhǐ shēngchǎn yìlièbiàn cáiliào héchá】**
virtual nuclear test The numerical simulation of a nuclear explosion test done by advanced computer programs and high performance computers. (Modified from: Reference [2], p430)	**虚拟核试验【xūnǐ héshìyàn】** 用先进的计算机程序和高性能计算机对核爆试验进行数值模拟。(改自：参考文献[2]，p430)
visual observation	**目视观察【mùshì guānchá】**
voluntary offer agreement	**自愿提交协定【zìyuàn tíjiāo xiédìng】**
voluntary reporting scheme on nuclear material and specified equipment and non-nuclear material	**关于核材料、规定设备和非核材料自愿报告机制【guānyú hécáiliào guīdìngshèbèi hé fēihécáiliào zìyuàn bàogào jīzhì】**
vulnerability assessment	**易损性评定【yìsǔnxìng píngdìng】**
waste from nuclear fuel cycle	**核燃料循环废物【héránliào xúnhuán fèiwù】**
waste from nuclear power plant	**核电厂废物【hédiànchǎng fèiwù】**
waste solidification	**废物固化【fèiwù gùhuà】**
waste storage	**废物贮存【fèiwù zhùcún】**
weapon-grade plutonium Plutonium containing no more than 7% Pu-240. (From: Reference [1], p233)	**武器级钚【wǔqìjí bù】** 含小于或等于7%以下钚-240的钚。(源自：参考文献[1]，p233)

Note: Pu containing much more than 7% Pu-240 can actually be used in a nuclear weapon. (From: Reference [13], p32-33)	注：含远大于 7%以上钚-240 的钚事实上亦可用于核武器。(源自：参考文献[13]，p32-33)
weapon-grade uranium Enriched uranium containing no less than 90% U-235. (From: Reference [1], p233)	**武器级铀【wǔqìjí yóu】** 含大于或等于 90%以上铀-235 的铀。(源自：参考文献[1]，p233)
weaponization	**武器化【wǔqìhuà】**
weaponization of space To deploy systems or components specifically designed to fight a war in or from space, or military capabilities on the earth specifically designed to destroy or disable targets in space. (Modified From: Reference [56], p29) Refer to "**militarization of space**"	**外空武器化【wàikōng wǔqìhuà】** 部署专门设计用于在/从外空作战的系统或部件，或部署专门设计用于在地球上攻击外空中目标的军事能力。(改自：参考文献[56]，p29) 参见"**外空军事化**"
weapon-usable material	**可用于武器的材料** **【kěyòngyú wǔqì de cáiliào】**
Western Group	**西方国家集团** **【xīfāng guójiā jítuán】**
wet storage	**湿法贮存【shīfǎ zhùcún】**
X-ray laser pumped by nuclear explosion	**核爆激励 X 射线激光器** **【hébào jīlì X shèxiàn jīguāngqì】**
yellow cake A concentrate produced during the uranium milling process that contains about 80% U_3O_8 with small amounts of uranyl salts. In preparation for uranium enrichment, the yellowcake is converted to uranium hexafluoride gas (UF_6). In the preparation of natural uranium reactor fuel, yellowcake is processed into purified uranium dioxide. (From: Reference [12])	**黄饼【huángbǐng】** 铀水冶过程中的中间产物，含有大约 80％带着少量铀酰盐的八氧化三铀(U_3O_8)。用于铀浓缩的黄饼被转化成六氟化铀气体(UF_6)，用于天然铀反应堆燃料的黄饼被加工成纯净的二氧化铀。(源自：参考文献[12])

yield	威力【wēilì】
yield-to-weight ratio	比威力【bǐwēilì】
Zangger Committee The Zangger Committee, also known as the Nuclear Non-proliferation Treaty Exporters Committee, is a nuclear export group, which consists of parties of the Nuclear Non-proliferation Treaty (NPT) who have the capability of nuclear export. The committee was formed in 1971. It aims to prevent the prohibition of nuclear weapons by controlling the export of nuclear materials and equipment from parties of the NPT to non-nuclear-weapon states. The main export control mechanism of the committee is the "Trigger List". Items on this List exported to non-nuclear- weapon states must be subject to IAEA safeguards. The committee now has 36 member states. (Modified from: Reference [1], p374)	桑戈委员会【sānggē wěiyuánhuì】 一些有核出口能力的《不扩散核武器条约》(NPT)缔约国组成的核出口控制集团，又称 NPT 出口国委员会。该委员会于 1971 年成立，宗旨是控制《不扩散核武器条约》成员国对没有核武器的非条约成员国的核材料和核设备的出口，以防止核武器扩散。委员会的主要出口控制机制是“触发清单”，即向无核武器国家出口触发清单上的项目，接收国必须接受“国际原子能机构”的保障监督。目前该委员会有 36 个成员国。(改自：参考文献[1]，p374)
Zangger Committee Export Guidelines	桑戈委员会出口准则 【sānggē wěiyuánhuì chūkǒu zhǔnzé】
zero-yield experiment Refer to "**subcritical experiment**"	零威力实验【língwēilì shíyàn】 参见“次临界实验”

ABBREVIATIONS

ABM Treaty	**Treaty Between the United States of America and the Union of Soviet Republics on the Limitation of Anti-ballistic Missile Systems**	美苏关于限制反弹道导弹系统条约(反导条约)
AF&F	**Arming, Fuzing & Firing system**	引控系统
ASC Program	**Advanced Simulation and Computing Program**	先进模拟与计算计划
ASCI	**Accelerated Strategic Computing Initiative**	加速战略计算倡议
ASEAN	**Association of Southeast Asian Nations**	东盟
BWR	**Boiling Water Reactor**	沸水堆
C3I	**Command, Control, Communication & Intelligence**	指挥、控制、通信和情报系统(C3I 系统)
C4I	**Command, Control, Communications, Computing & Intelligence**	指挥、控制、通信、计算和情报系统(C4I 系统)
CCD	**Conference of the Committee on Disarmament**	裁军委员会会议
CD	**Conference on Disarmament**	裁军谈判会议
CEP	**Circular Error Probable**	圆概率偏差
CORRTEX	**Continuous Reflectometry for Radius vs Time Experiment**	科尔太克斯法
CSA	**Canned Subassembly**	罐装组件
CSA	**Comprehensive Safeguards Agreement**	全面保障监督协定
CSBMs	**Confidence and Security Building**	建立信任与安全

	Measures	措施
CTBT	**Comprehensive Test Ban Treaty**	全面禁止核试验条约
DA	**Destructive Analysis**	破坏性分析
DIV	**Design Information Verification**	设计资料核查
DUPIC	**Direct Use of Spent PWR Fuel in CANDU Reactors Process**	杜皮克工艺
EEL	**Essential Equipment List**	重要设备清单
ELINT	**electronic intelligence**	电子情报
ENCD	**Eighteen-Nation Committee on Disarmament**	十八国裁军委员会
HEU	**High-Enriched Uranium**	高浓铀
HTGR	**High Temperature Gas-Cooled Reactor**	高温气冷堆
HWR	**Heavy Water Reactor**	重水堆
IAEA	**International Atomic Energy Agency**	国际原子能机构
ICF	**Inertial Confinement Fusion**	惯性约束聚变
IDC	**International Data Center**	国际数据中心
IMO	**International Maritime Organization**	国际海事组织
IMS	**International Monitoring System**	国际监测系统
INF Treaty	**Treaty Between the United States of America and the Union of Soviet Socialist Republics on the Elimination of Their Intermediate-Range and Shorter-Range Missiles**	美苏关于消除两国中程及中短程导弹条约(中导条约)
INFCIRC	**Information Circular**	信息通报

IW	**Information Warfare**	信息战
KMP	**Key Measurement Point**	关键测量点
LEU	**Low-Enriched Uranium**	低浓铀
LOF	**Location Outside Facilities**	设施外场所
LOW	**Launch-on-Warning**	预警即发射
LUA	**Launch-under-Attack**	遇袭即发射
LWR	**Light Water Reactor**	轻水堆
MAD	**Mutual Assured Destruction**	相互确保摧毁
MaRV	**Maneuverable Reentry Vehicle**	机动再入弹头
MBA	**Material Balance Area**	核材料平衡区
MBP	**Material Balance Period**	材料平衡周期
MIRV	**Multiple Independently Targetable Reentry Vehicle**	分导式多弹头
MNSR	**Miniature Neutron Source Reactor**	微型中子源反应堆
MOX	**Mixed Oxide**	混合氧化物
MTCR	**Missile Technology Control Regime**	导弹技术控制制度
MUF	**Material Unaccounted For**	不明材料量
NEM	**Nuclear-Explosive Material**	核爆材料
NEMP	**Nuclear Electromagnetic Pulse**	核电磁脉冲
NIF	**National Ignition Facility**	国家点火装置
NNWS	**Non-Nuclear Weapon State**	无核武器国家
NPT	**Treaty on the Non-Proliferation of Nuclear Weapons**	不扩散核武器条约

NSG	**Nuclear Suppliers Group**	核供应国集团
NTMs	**National Technical Means**	国家技术手段
NTS	**Nuclear Threshold State**	核门槛国家
NWS	**Nuclear Weapon State**	核武器国家
OSCE	**Organization for Security and Cooperation in Europe**	欧洲安全与合作组织
OSI	**on-site inspection**	现场视察
PAL	**Permissive Action Link**	密码锁(亦称启动连接装置)
PNE	**Treaty Between the United States of America and the Union of Soviet Socialist Republics on Underground Nuclear Explosion for Peaceful Purposes**	美苏和平利用地下核爆炸条约
PTBT	**Treaty Banning Nuclear Weapon Tests in the Atmosphere, in Outer Space and Under Water**	禁止在大气层、外层空间和水下进行核武器试验条约
PUREX Process	**Plutonium Uranium Recovery by Extraction Process**	普雷克斯流程
PWR	**Pressurized Water Reactor**	压水堆
RDD	**Radioactive Dispersal Device**	放射性物质散布装置
RMA	**Revolution in Military Affairs**	军事变革
RRRW	**Reduced Residual Radioactivity Weapon**	弱剩余放射性武器(3R 弹)
RSAC	**Regional System of Accounting for and Control of Nuclear Material**	地区核材料衡算和控制系统
SALT II	**Treaty Between the United States of**	美苏限制进攻性

Treaty	**America and the Union of Soviet Socialist Republics on the Limitation of Strategic Offensive Arms**	战略武器条约
SALT I	**Interim Agreement Between the United States of America and the Union of Soviet Socialist Republics on Certain Measures with Respect to the Limitation of Strategic Offensive Arms**	美苏限制进攻性战略武器的某些措施的临时协定
SAR	**Synthetic Aperture Radar**	合成孔径雷达
SDI	**Strategic Defense Initiative**	战略防御倡议
SORT	**Treaty Between the United States of American and the Russian Federation On Strategic Offensive Reductions**	美俄削减进攻性战略武器条约(莫斯科条约)
SQ	**Significant Quantity**	重要量
SQP	**Small Quantities Protocol**	小数量议定书
SRD	**Shipper/Receiver Difference**	发方/收方差额
SSAC	**State System of Accounting for and Control of Nuclear Material**	国家核材料衡算和控制系统
START I	**Treaty Between the United States of America and the Union of Soviet Socialist Republics on the Reduction and Limitation of Offensive Strategic Arms**	美苏关于削减和限制进攻性战略武器条约
START II	**Treaty Between the United States of America and the Russian Federation on Further Reduction and Limitation of Strategic Offensive Arms**	美俄关于进一步削减和限制进攻性战略武器条约
THOREX Process	**Thorium Extraction Process**	梭雷克斯流程
TNCD	**Ten-Nation Committee on Disarmament**	十国裁军委员会

TTBT	**Treaty Between the United States of America and the Union of Soviet Socialist Republics on the Limitation of Underground Nuclear Weapon Tests**	美苏限制地下核武器试验条约(限当量条约)
UNDC	**United Nations Disarmament Commission**	联合国裁军审议委员会
UNIDIR	**United Nations Institute for Disarmament Research**	联合国裁军研究所
V&V	**verification and validation**	验证与确认

REFERENCES

[1] 刘华秋 主编. 军备控制与裁军手册[M]. 北京: 国防工业出版社, 2000.
Liu Huaqiu. Arms Control and Disarmament Handbook. Beijing: National Defense Industry Press, 2000.

[2] 国防科技名词大典——核能卷编委会. 国防科技名词大典——核能卷[M]. 北京: 航空工业出版社, 兵器工业出版社, 原子能出版社, 2002.
Edit Committee of National Defense Science and Technology Dictionary——Nuclear Energy Column. National Defense Science and Technology Dictionary——Nuclear Energy. Beijing: Aviation Industry Press, Enginery Industry Press, Atomic Energy Press, 2002.

[3] 中国军事百科全书编审委员会. 中国军事百科全书(第 5, 6 卷)[M]. 北京: 军事科学出版社, 1997.
Edit Committee for Chinese Military Encyclopedia. Chinese Military Encyclopedia (Volume 5, 6). Beijing: Military Science Press, 1997.

[4] 国际原子能机构(IAEA). 国际原子能机构保障监督术语[M/OL]//国际核查丛书 (2001 版)[M]. 维也纳: IAEA, 2002.
International Atomic Energy Agency (IAEA). IAEA Safeguards Glossary 2001 Edition. International Nuclear Verification Series No.3. Vienna: IAEA, 2002. Available as of March 2008 at:
http://www-pub.iaea.org/MTCD/publications/PDF/nvs-3-cd/PDF/NVS3_scr.pdf

[5] 北大西洋公约组织(NATO). 北约英俄核术语词典[M/OL]. 北约, 2007.
North Atlantic Treaty Organization. NATO English and Russian Nuclear Terms. NATO, 2007. Available as of March 2008 at:
http://www.nato.int/docu/glossary/eng-nuclear/nuc_glos-e.pdf

[6] Shelkh Ali. 和平与核战争词典[M]. Santa Barbara, CA: ABC-Clio 信息部, 1989.
Sheikh Ali. The Peace and Nuclear War Dictionary. Santa Barbara, CA: ABC-Clio Information Services, 1989.

[7] 国家科学院国际安全和军控委员会(CISAC). 美国未来核武器政策[M/OL]. 华盛顿特区: 国家科学院出版社, 1997.
Committee on International Security and Arms Control (CISAC) of the National Academy of Sciences. The Future of U.S. Nuclear Weapons Policy, Washington, D.C.: The National Academies Press, 1997. Available as of March 2008 at: http://www.nap.edu/catalog.php?record_id=5796

[8] 美国国务院. 军控与裁军术语表[M/OL].

U.S. Department of State: Arms Control and Disarmament Glossary of Terms. Available as of March 2008 at: http://usinfo.state.gov/is/Archive_Index/Arms_Control_and_Disarmament_Glossary_of_Terms.html

[9] 美国国防部, 参谋长联席会议. 国防部军事及相关术语词典[M/OL]. 2007.
Department of Defense, Joint Chiefs of Staff. Department of Defense Dictionary of Military and Associated Terms, 1-02. 2007. Available as of March 2008 at: http://www.dtic.mil/doctrine/jel/new_pubs/jp1_02.pdf or http://www.dtic.mil/doctrine/jel/doddict

[10] Rene Bierbaum 等. 能源部核武器可靠性定义: 历史, 描述和执行[R/OL]. 圣地亚国家实验室, SAND99-8240 报告, 1999.
Rene Bierbaum, et al. DOE Nuclear Weapon Reliability Definition: History, Description, and Implementation. Sandia National Laboratories, report SAND99-8240, 1999. Available as of March 2008 at: http://www.osti.gov/bridge/purl.cover.jsp?purl=/6105-eS62Sb/webviewable/ or http://www.osti.gov/bridge/servlets/purl/6105-eS62Sb/webviewable/6105.PDF

[11] 国家科学院国际安全和军控委员会(CISAC). 监察核武器及核爆材料: 方法与能力评估[R/OL]. 华盛顿特区: 国家学院出版社, 2005.
Committee on International Security and Arms Control (CISAC) of the National Academy of Sciences. Monitoring Nuclear Weapons and Nuclear-Explosive Materials: An Assessment of Methods and Capabilities. Washington, D.C.: The National Academies Press, 2005. Available as of March 2008 at: http://www.nap.edu/catalog.php?record_id=11265

[12] 科学与国际安全研究所 (ISIS) . ISIS 非法采购网络的案例研究, 电子书术语[M/OL]. 2003.
Institute for Science and International Security (ISIS). ISIS Case Studies of Illicit Procurement Networks, E-Book Glossary, 2003. Available as of March 2008 at: http://www.exportcontrols.org/glossary.html

[13] 国家科学院国际安全和军控委员会(CISAC). 管理和控制剩余的武器级钚[M/OL]. 华盛顿特区: 国家学院出版社, 1994.
Committee on International Security and Arms Control (CISAC) of the National Academy of Sciences. The Management and Disposition of Excess Weapons Plutonium. Washington D.C.: The National Academies Press, 1994. Available as of March 2008 at: http://www.nap.edu/catalog.php?record_id=2345

[14] 国际原子能机构(IAEA). 国家核燃料循环概况[M/OL]. 技术报告序列号 No.404.

维也纳, IAEA, 2001.
International Atomic Energy Agency (IAEA). Country Nuclear Fuel Cycle Profiles. Technical Reports Series No.404, Vienna: IAEA, 2001. Available as of March 2008 at:
http://www-pub.iaea.org/MTCD/publications/PDF/TRS404_scr.pdf

[15] 国际原子能机构(IAEA). 国际原子能机构与《不扩散核武器条约》有关国家之间协议的框架和内容. INFIRCIR/153 协议, 奥地利: IAEA, 1972.
International Atomic Energy Agency (IAEA).The Structure and Content of Agreements Between the Agency and States Required in Connection with the Treaty on the Non-Proliferation of Nuclear Weapons. IAEA INFCIRC/153. Austria: IAEA, 1972. Available as of March 2008 at:
http://www.iaea.org/Publications/Documents/Infcircs/Others/infcirc153.pdf

[16] 联合国裁军研究所(裁研所)和核查、研究、培训和信息中心(核查). 安全术语: 核查与遵约手册[M]. 瑞士・日内瓦: 联合国裁军研究所(UNIDIR); 英国・伦敦: 核查研究、培训和信息中心(VERTIC). UNDIR/2003/10.
United Nations Institute for Disarmament Research (UNIDIR) and The Verification Research, Training and Information Centre (VERTIC). Coming to Terms with Security: A Handbook on Verification and Compliance. Geneva, Switzerland and London, United Kingdom: UNIDIR and VERTIC, 2003. UNIDIR/2003/10.

[17] 罗纳德・里根. 关于国家安全的全国讲话[R/OL]. [1983-03-23].
Ronald Reagan. Address to the Nation on National Security. March 23, 1983. Available as of March 2008 at:
http://www.globalsecurity.org/space/library/congress/1996_cr/s960329a.htm

[18] 王文荣. 战略学[M]. 北京: 国防大学出版社, 1999.
Wang Wenrong. Science of Military Strategy. Beijing: National Defense University Press, 1999.

[19] Steven Tulliu, Thomas Schmalberger. 安全术语: 军控、裁军和建立信任措施词典[M/OL]. 日内瓦: 联合国裁军研究所. UNDIR/2003/22.
Steven Tulliu and Thomas Schmalberger. Coming To Terms with Security: A Lexicon for Arms Control, Disarmament and Confidence Building. Geneva: United Nations Institute for Disarmament Research, 2003. UNDIR/2003/22. Available as of March 2008 at:
http://www.unidir.ch/pdf/ouvrages/pdf-1-92-9045-156-4-en.pdf

[20] William Graham 等. 评估电磁脉冲攻击对美国的威胁的委员会报告[R/OL]. 公

共法, 2004: 106-398.

William Graham et al. Report of the Commission to Assess the Threat to the United States from Electromagnetic Pulse (EMP) Attack. 2004. Public Law 106-398. Available as of March 2008 at: http://www.globalsecurity.org/wmd/library/congress/2004_r/04-07-22emp.pdf

[21] 美国国防部. 四年一度防务评估[R/OL]. 国防部, 2006.

亦见: Charles Lutes. 威慑能定制吗? 无限制战争讨论会年报[R/OL]. Johns Hopkins 大学应用物理实验室, 2007.

Department of Defense. The Quadrennial Defense Review. Department of Defense, February 2006. Available as of March 2008 at: http://www.defenselink.mil/pubs/pdfs/QDR20060203.pdf.

See also: Charles Lutes. Can Deterrence Be Tailored? Unrestricted Warfare Symposium Proceedings 2007. Johns Hopkins University Applied Physics Laboratory. Available as of March 2008 at: http://www.jhuapl.edu/urw_symposium/previous/2007/pages/proceedings/2007/papers/Lutes.pdf

[22] Keir Lieber , Daryl Press. 美国核优势的升起[J]. 外交事务, 2006, 3 月－4 月.

Keir Lieber and Daryl Press. The Rise of U.S. Nuclear Primacy. Foreign Affairs, March/April 2006. Available as of March 2008 at: http://www.foreignaffairs.org/20060301faessay85204/keir-a-lieber-daryl-g-press/the-rise-of-u-s-nuclear-primacy.html

[23] Thomas Schelling. 军备及影响[M]. New Haven, CT: 耶鲁大学出版社, 1966.

Thomas Schelling. Arms and Influence. New Haven, CT: Yale University Press, 1966.

[24] Peter Gizewski. 世界新秩序中的最低核威慑[C]//极光论文(24). 渥太华: 加拿大全球安全中心, 1994.

Peter Gizewski. Minimum Nuclear Deterrence in a New World Order. Aurora Papers No. 24. Ottawa: Canadian Centre for Global Security, 1994.

[25] 中华人民共和国核出口管制条例 (修订版)[M]. 2001.

Regulations of the People's Republic of China on the Control of Nuclear Export. Revised Edition. 2001.

[26] 连培生. 原子能工业(修订版)[M]. 北京: 原子能出版社, 2002.

Lian Peisheng. Atomic Energy Industry (Revised Edition). Beijing: Atomic Energy Press, 2002.

[27] Lynn Eden 和 Steven Miller, eds. 核问题辩论: 对战略核武器与军备控制争论的理解[M]. 纽约: 康奈尔大学出版社, 1989.
Lynn Eden and Steven Miller, eds. Nuclear Arguments: Understanding the Strategic Nuclear Arms and Arms Control Debates. New York: Cornell University Press, 1989.

[28] John Baylis 等. 现代战略 I : 理论和概念(Phil Williams, "危机管理"部分)[M]. 伦敦和悉尼: Croom Helm 出版社, 1987.
Phil Williams. Crisis Management. In: John Baylis et al. Contemporary Strategy I: Theories and Concepts. London and Sydney: Croom Helm, 1987.

[29] 北大西洋公约组织(NATO). 非北约核术语和定义词汇表[M]//北约—俄罗斯核术语和定义词汇表, 附录 2[M/OL]. NATO, 2007.
North Atlantic Treaty Organization(NATO). NATO-Russia Glossary of Nuclear Terms and Definitions. Appendix 2: Non-NATO Nuclear Terms and Definitions. NATO, 2007. Available as of March 2008 at:
http://www.nato.int/docu/glossary/eng-nuclear/nuc_glos-e.pdf

[30] Robert Thorn, Donald Westervelt. 流体核试验[R], LA-10902-MS UC-2. 洛斯·阿拉莫斯: 洛斯·阿拉莫斯国家实验室, 1987.
Robert Thorn and Donald Westervelt. Hydronuclear Experiments, LA-10902-MS UC-2. Los Alamos: Los Alamos National Laboratory, 1987.

[31] 彭广谦 等著. 战略学[M]. 北京: 军事科学院出版, 2001.
Peng Guangqian et al. Science of Military Strategy. Beijing: Academy of Military Sciences Press, 2001.

[32] Hangbok Choi 等. DUPIC 燃料兼容性分析进展 - I: 反应堆物理[J]. 核技术, 2006, 153(1).
Hangbok Choi et al. Progress of the DUPIC Fuel Compatibility Analysis - I: Reactor Physics. Nuclear Technology, 2006, 153 (1).

[33] 王厚卿, 张兴业. 战役学[M]. 北京: 国防大学出版社, 2000.
Wang Houqing, Zhang Xingye. Science of Campaign. Beijing: National Defense University, 2000.

[34] 中华人民共和国. 2006 年中国的国防[M/OL]. 中华人民共和国国务院新闻办公室. 北京. [2006-12].
People's Republic of China. China's National Defense in 2006. Information Office of the State Council of the People's Republic of China. Beijing: December 2006. Available as of March 2008 at:
http://www.chinadaily.com.cn/china/2006-12/29/content_771191.htm

[35] 1978 年核不扩散法案[M]. 公共法. 1978, 95-242.

Nuclear Non-Proliferation Act of 1978, Public Law 95-242. Available as of March 2008 at: http://www.nti.org/db/china/engdocs/nnpa1978.htm

[36] 中国军事网. 中国人手里会没有“杀手锏”吗? [EB/OL].

China Military Net. Could the Chinese be Without "Assassin's Mace" in Hands? Available as of March 2008 at: http://military.china.com/zh_cn/critical3/27/20060216/13099404.html

[37] 洛斯・阿拉莫斯国家实验室. NNSA 先进的模拟和计算程序[CP/OL].

Los Alamos National Laboratory. NNSA Advanced Simulation and Computing Program Website. Available as of March 2008 at: http://www.lanl.gov/projects/asci/

[38] 人民网. 中国建立法制化防扩散出口管制体系[EB/OL]. [2003-12-04].

People Net. China's Established Legal Systems for Non-proliferation and Export Controls. December 4, 2003. Available as of March 2008 at: http://www.people.com.cn/GB/junshi/1076/2227410.html

[39] Jamie Ann Calabrese . 胡萝卜还是大棒?利比亚和美国针对无赖国家所做的努力[J/OL]. 战略观察, 2004, 3(11).

Jamie Ann Calabrese. Carrots or Sticks? Libya and U.S. Efforts to Influence Rogue States. Strategic Insights. Volume 3 (11), 2004. Available as of March 2008 at: https://www.maxwell.af.mil/au/awc/awcgate/nps/ccc_calabrese_nov04.pdf

[40] 美国国务院. 凯南及围堵政策[M/OL]. 1947.

U.S. Department of State. Kennan and Containment, 1947. Available as of March 2008 at: http://www.state.gov/r/pa/ho/time/cwr/17601.htm

[41] David Yost. 劝阻和盟国[J/OL]. 战略观察, 2005, 4 (2).

David Yost. Dissuasion and Allies. Strategic Insights. 2005, 4 (2). Available as of March 2008 at: http://www.ccc.nps.navy.mil/si/2005/Feb/yostfeb05.asp

[42] 美国国务院. 八国集团.

U.S. Department of State. The G-8 Global Partnership. Available as of March 2008 at: http://www.state.gov/t/isn/c12743.htm

[43] 2006 俄罗斯联邦任期八国集团官方网站. 八国集团历史.

Official Website of the G-8 Presidency of the Russian Federation in 2006. G-8 History. Available as of March 2008 at: http://en.g8russia.ru/g8/history/shortinfo/

R

[44] 情况说明书: 对核恐怖主义作战的全球计划.
The Global Initiative to Combat Nuclear Terrorism. Fact Sheet. Available as of March 2008 at:
http://www.whitehouse.gov/news/releases/2006/07/print/20060715-3.html

[45] Sara Wood. 有官员称，平衡对中美关系至关重要. 美国军方新闻部. [2006-03-17].
Sara Wood. Balance Critical to U.S.-China Relationship, Officials Say. American Forces Press Service, March 17, 2006. Available as of March 2008 at: http://www.defenselink.mil/news/newsarticle.aspx?id=15136

[46] Alastair Iain Johnston. 中国新的"旧思维" [J]. 国际安全, 1995/1996, 20(3).
Alastair Iain Johnston. China's New "Old Thinking". International Security, 1995/96, 20 (3).

[47] 核供应集团(NSG)网站.
The Nuclear Suppliers Group (NSG) Website. Available as of March 2008 at:
http://www.nuclearsuppliersgroup.org/

[48] 美国国会图书馆, 联邦政府研究部. 苏联术语表[M]//国家研究地域手册丛书[M/OL].
Library of Congress. Federal Research Division, Countries Studies Area Handbook Series, Glossary - Soviet Union. Available as of March 2008 at:
http://lcweb2.loc.gov/frd/cs/soviet_union/su_glos.html

[49] 北大西洋公约组织(NATO). 北约和北约一俄罗斯核术语和定义[M] //北约一俄罗斯核术语和定义词汇表, 附录 1[M/OL]. NATO, 2007.
North Atlantic Treaty Organization. NATO-Russia Glossary of Nuclear Terms and Definitions. Appendix 1: NATO and NATO-Russia Nuclear Terms and Definitions. NATO, 2007. Available as of March 2008 at:
http://www.nato.int/docu/glossary/eng-nuclear/

[50] 美国国防部. 美国国防部合作减少威胁(CTR)计划网站[EB/OL]. 1998.
Department of Defense. Department of Defense Cooperative Threat Reduction (CTR) Program Website,1998. Available as of March 2008 at:
http://www.dod.mil/pubs/ctr/instability.html

[51] 国际原子能机构(IAEA). IAEA 保障监督: 防止核武器扩散[EB/OL]. 新闻通告. 2002.
International Atomic Energy Agency (IAEA). IAEA Safeguards: Stemming the Spread of Nuclear Weapons. Factsheet. 2002. Available as of March 2008 at:
http://www.iaea.org/Publications/Factsheets/English/S1_Safeguards.pdf

R

[52] 新华网. 核材料实物保护公约: 加强对核设施核材料保护[EB/OL]. [2005-07-08].
Xinhua Net. Convention on the Physical Protection of Nuclear Material: Enhancing Physical Protection of Nuclear Material and Facilities. Xinhua Net. July 8, 2005. Available as of March 2008 at:
http://news.xinhuanet.com/world/2005-07/09/content_3195596.htm

[53] 中华人民共和国驻印度大使. 记者招待会: 和平共处五项基本原则. 和平共处五项基本原则提出 50 周年纪念[EB/OL]. [2004-06-14].
Embassy of the People's Republic of China in India. Backgrounder: Five Principles of Peaceful Coexistence. The 50th Anniversary of the Initiation of the Five Principles of Peaceful Co-Existence. June 14 2004. Available as of March 2008 at: http://in.china-embassy.org/eng/ssygd/fiveprinciple/t132640.htm

[54] 联合国裁军研究所(裁研所)和核查、研究、培训和信息中心(核查). 关键术语[M]// 安全术语: 核查与遵约手册[M/OL]. 瑞士日内瓦和英国伦敦: UNIDIR 和 VERTIC. 2003.
United Nations Institute for Disarmament Research (UNIDIR) and The Verification Research, Training and Information Centre (VERTIC). Coming to Terms with Security: A Handbook on Verification and Compliance. Key Terms. Geneva, Switzerland and London, United Kingdom: UNIDIR and VERTIC, 2003. Available as of March 2008 at:
http://www.unidir.org/pdf/articles/pdf-art1980.pdf

[55] Steven Lambakis. 重新审议非对称战争[J]. 联合军力季刊, 2005, (36).
Steven Lambakis. Reconsidering Asymmetric Warfare. Joint Force Quarterly, 2005, (36). Available as of March 2008 at:
http://www.dtic.mil/doctrine/jel/jfq_pubs/1736.pdf

[56] Michael Krepon, Christopher Clary. 确保外空还是统治外空? 反对外空武器化的案例[M]. 华盛顿特区: Henry L. Stimson 中心, 2003.
Michael Krepon with Christopher Clary. Space Assurance or Space Dominance? The Case Against Weaponizing Space. Washington, D.C.: The Henry L. Stimson Center, 2003. Available as of March 2008 at:
http://www.stimson.org/wos/pdf/space2.pdf

[57] Celeste Wallander. 得与失: 戈尔巴乔夫的"新思维"[J]. 华盛顿季刊, 2002, 25(1).
Celeste Wallander. Lost and Found: Gorbachev's "New Thinking". The Washington Quarterly, 2002, 25 (1). Available as of March 2008 at:
http://www.twq.com/02winter/wallander.pdf

[58] Matthew Evangelista. 非武装力量：结束冷战的跨国努力[M]. 纽约伊萨卡：康内尔大学出版社, 1999.

Matthew Evangelista. Unarmed Forces: The Transnational Effort to End the Cold War. Ithaca, N.Y.: Cornell University Press, 1999.

[59] 国家科学院国际安全和军控委员会(CISAC). 有关“全面禁止核试验条约”批准的技术问题[M/OL]. 华盛顿特区：国家学院出版社, 2002.

Committee on International Security and Arms Control (CISAC) of the National Academy of Sciences. Technical Issues Related to Ratification of the Comprehensive Nuclear Test Ban Treaty. Washington, D.C.: The National Academies Press, 2002. Available as of March 2008 at: http://www.nap.edu/catalog.php?record_id=10471

[60] 美国国防部部长副助理核问题办公室. 核武器确信性.

Office to the Deputy Assistant to the Secretary of Defense for Nuclear Matters. Nuclear Weapons Surety. Available as of March 2008 at: http://www.acq.osd.mil/ncbdp/nm/nuclearweaponssurety.html

[61] 美国陆军司令部. 战场手册(No.1)[M/OL]. 华盛顿特区：陆军部, 2005.

U.S. Department of the Army. Field Manual No.1. Washington D.C.: Department of the Army, 2005. Available as of March 2008 at: http://www.army.mil/fm1/chapter3.html

[62] Albert Latter, Ernest Martinelli. 主动和被动防御[EB/OL]. 1965.

Albert Latter and Ernest Martinelli. Active and Passive Defense, 1965. Available as of March 2008 at: http://stinet.dtic.mil/cgi-bin/GetTRDoc?AD=AD676973&Location=U2&doc=GetTRDoc.pdf

[63] Martin Pilch 等. 圣地亚 ASCI 验证与确认计划的指导方针一内容与形式：版本 2.0[R/OL]. SAND2000-3101, 非限制发行, 2001.

Martin Pilch, et al. Guidelines for Sandia ASCI Verification and Validation Plans - Content and Format: Version 2.0. SAND2000-3101, Unlimited Distribution, 2001. Available as of March 2008 at: http://www.prod.sandia.gov/cgi-bin/techlib/access-control.pl/2000/003101.pdf

[64] 戈尔巴乔夫. 诺贝尔演讲[R/OL]. [1991-06-05].

Mikhail Gorbachev. Nobel Lecture. June 5, 1991. Available as of March 2008 at: http://nobelprize.org/nobel_prizes/peace/laureates/1990/gorbachev-lecture.html

[65] Gareth Evans. 第 48 界联合国大会第五次全体会议上的讲话[R/OL]. [1993-9-27].
Gareth Evans. Speech to the 5th Plenary Meeting of the 48th Session of the United Nations General Assembly. September 27, 1993. Available as of March 2008 at:
http://www.crisisgroup.org/library/documents/speeches_ge/foreign_minister/1993/270993_fm_uncooperatingforpeaces.pdf

[66] Douglas Feith. 国防部副部长 Douglas J. Feith 关于政策的讲话[C]//参议院军事事务听证会听取《核态势评估》报告[R/OL]. [2002-02-14].
Douglas Feith. Statement of the Honorable Douglas J. Feith, Undersecretary of Defense for Policy, Senate Armed Services Hearing on the Nuclear Posture Review. February 14, 2002. Available as of March 2008 at:
http://armed-services.senate.gov/statement/2002/Feith.pdf

[67] 美国国防部. 美国核态势评估(摘录)[R]. 2001 年 12 月 31 日递交. 美国国防部, [2002-01-08].
Department of Defense. U.S. Nuclear Posture Review (Excerpts). Submitted to Congress on December 31, 2001. Department of Defense. January 8, 2002. Available as of March 2008 at:
http://www.globalsecurity.org/wmd/library/policy/dod/npr.htm.

[68] Linton Brooks. Linton F. Brooks 大使(美国能源部副部长、国家核安全管理局局长)在众议院武装力量委员会战略力量分委会上的陈述[R/OL]. [2006-03-01].
Linton Brooks. Statement of Ambassador Linton F. Brooks, Under Secretary for Nuclear Security and Administrator, National Nuclear Security Administration U.S. Department of Energy Before the House Armed Services Committee Subcommittee on Strategic Forces. March 1, 2006. Available as of March 2008 at:
http://www.nipp.org/Adobe/RRW%20final%20with%20foreword%207.30.07.pdf

[69] Gregory Giles 等. 最低核威慑研究: 最终报告[R/OL]. 国防部减小威胁局先进系统与概念办公室. [2003-05-15].
Gregory Giles et al. Minimum Nuclear Deterrence Research: Final Report. Advanced Systems and Concepts Office, Defense Threat Reduction Agency. May 15, 2003. Available as of March 2008 at:
http://www.dtra.mil/documents/asco/publications/MinimumNuclearDeterrencePhase2.pdf

[70] 王仲春. 核武器核国家核战略[M]. 北京: 时事出版社, 2007.

Wang Zhongchun. Nuclear Weapons, Nuclear States, Nuclear Strategy. Beijing: Current Events Publishing House, 2007.

[71] 美国技术评估办公室. 威慑、美国核战略和弹道导弹防御[J]. 弹道导弹防御技术, 1985.

U.S. Office of Technology Assessment. Deterrence, U.S. Nuclear Strategy, and BMD. Ballistic Missile Defense Technologies. 1985. Available as of March 2008 at: http://www.princeton.edu/~ota/disk2/1985/8504/8504.PDF

[72] James Russell, James Wirtz. 静悄悄的变革: 新的核三位一体[J/OL]. 战略观察 2002, 1 (3).

James Russell and James Wirtz. A Quiet Revolution: The New Nuclear Triad. Strategic Insights. 2002,1(3). Available as of March 2008 at: http://www.ccc.nps.navy.mil/si/may02/triad.asp

[73] 中华人民共和国国务院. 中华人民共和国核两用品及相关技术出口管制条例(修订版)[M/OL]. [2007-01-26].

The State Council of the People's Republic of China. Regulations of the People's Republic of China on Export Control of Dual-Use Nuclear Goods and the Related Technologies. Revised Edition. January 26, 2007. Available as of March 2008 at:
http://www.gov.cn/zwgk/2007-02/16/content_529172.htm

[74] 中华人民共和国国务院. 中华人民共和国核出口管制条例(修订版)[M/OL].

[2006-11-09]The State Council of the People's Republic of China. Regulations of the People's Republic of China on the Control of Nuclear Export. Revised Edition. November 9, 2006. Available as of March 2008 at
:http://www.gov.cn/zwgk/2006-12/01/content_459513.htm

汉英·英汉核安全术语

中美核安全术语编委会

中国人民争取和平与裁军协会
中国科学家军备控制小组

美国国家科学院
美国科学院
政策与全球事务所
国际安全与军备控制委员会

原子能出版社
北京
www.aep.com.cn

国家科学院出版社
华盛顿特区
www.nap.edu

原子能出版社

原子能出版社是中央一级专业出版社，成立于 1973 年，前身是 1959 年成立的中国科学院原子核科学委员会编辑委员会。原子能出版社隶属于中国核工业集团公司，主要编辑出版核领域的各类科学技术图书、期刊、教材以及相关领域的各类书籍和辞书。

* *

图书在版编目(CIP)数据

汉英/英汉核安全术语/中国人民争取和平与裁军协会，
美国国家科学院编著. —北京：原子能出版社，2008.4
ISBN 978-7-5022-4102-5

Ⅰ.汉… Ⅱ. ①中…②美… Ⅲ. 核工程-安全技术-术语-英、汉 Ⅳ. TL7-64

中国版本图书馆 CIP 数据核字 (2008) 第 038028 号

汉英/英汉核安全术语

出版发行	原子能出版社 (北京市海淀区阜成路 43 号　100037)
责任编辑	卫广刚　李代斌
印　　刷	绵阳市科学城曙光印刷厂
经　　销	全国新华书店
开　　本	787mm×1092mm　1/16
印　　张	17
字　　数	420 千字
版　　次	2008 年 4 月第 1 版　2008 年 4 月第 1 次印刷
书　　号	ISBN 978-7-5022-4102-5
印　　数	1—2000
定　　价	128.00 元

国家科学院出版社

国家科学院出版社成立于 20 世纪 80 年代早期，是美国科学院、美国工程院、医学院和国家研究委员会的官方出版社。国家科学院出版社现有雇员 75 名，拥有 10 个部门，它们是：行政部、图文部、设计部、编辑部、网络策划部、执行和仓储部、市场部、印刷部、生产部和影印部。

The project that is the subject of this report was approved by the Governing Board of the National Research Council, whose members are drawn from the councils of the National Academy of Sciences, the National Academy of Engineering, and the Institute of Medicine. The members of the committee responsible for the report were chosen for their special competences and with regard for appropriate balance.

This study was supported by Contract No. DE-AT01-06NA26358, TO #16 between the National Academy of Sciences and the U.S. Department of Energy. Any opinions, findings, conclusions, or recommendations expressed in this publication are those of the author(s) and do not necessarily reflect the views of the organizations or agencies that provided support for the project.

International Standard Book Number-13: 978-0-309-11931-3

International Standard Book Number-10: 0-309-11931-6

Additional copies of this report are available from the National Academies Press, 500 Fifth Street, N.W., Lockbox285, Washington, D.C. 20055; (800) 624-6242 or (202) 334-3313 (in the United States); Internet, http://www.nap.edu

中美核安全术语编委会

CSGAC 工作小组

组长	田东风博士	中国工程物理研究院
成员	胡思得院士	中国工程物理研究院
	竺家亨	北京应用物理与计算数学研究所
	史建斌	北京应用物理与计算数学研究所
	伍　钧博士	北京应用物理与计算数学研究所
	余小玲	中国科学家军备控制小组
	何毅丹	中国科学家军备控制小组
	康春梅	中国工程物理研究院
	孙向丽博士	北京应用物理与计算数学研究所
	田景梅博士	北京应用物理与计算数学研究所

CISAC 工作小组

组长	**Ming-Shih Lu** 博士	布鲁克海文国家实验室，退休
成员	**Richard L. Garwin** 博士	IBM 公司华生研究中心，荣誉退休
	Raymond Jeanloz 博士	加利福尼亚大学伯克利分校
	Alastair Iain Johnston 博士	哈佛大学
	Alvin W. Trivelpiece 博士	橡树岭国家实验室，退休
职员	**Benjamin J. Rusek**	国际安全与军备控制委员会高级项目人员
	Anne Harrington	国际安全与军备控制委员会主任

中国人民争取和平与裁军协会

中国人民争取和平与裁军协会 (以下简称“**和裁会**”)是中国最大的民间和平组织，1985 年 6 月由国内有关人民团体和各界知名人士发起成立，目前共有 24 个重要的会员组织。

和裁会的宗旨是增进中国人民同世界各国人民的相互了解、友谊与合作，共同维护世界和平，反对军备竞赛和战争，要求实现军备控制和裁军，争取全面禁止和彻底销毁核武器及其他大规模杀伤性武器，保护生态环境，促进经济发展，推动社会进步。

和裁会已与全世界近 90 个国家约 300 个从事军控与裁军、全球和地区安全问题研究的民间和平组织和学术机构建立了不同形式的友好关系，开展各种交流与合作。

和裁会积极从事有关军控、裁军、和平与安全等问题的研究，每年都主办或合办国际学术研讨会，派专家学者出席各种国际会议和学术研讨会，接待外国代表团。

和裁会享有联合国经社理事会咨商地位，是联合国非政府组织大会的正式成员。

美国国家科学院——为国家提供科学、工程和医学咨询的机构

美国科学院是一个非盈利性民间机构，具有悠久的历史，拥有众多从事科学和工程研究的著名学者，致力于推进科技发展及运用科技为人类谋福利。根据国会 1863 年通过的宪章，授权科学院为联邦政府提供科学技术方面的咨询意见。拉尔夫·塞西隆博士是美国科学院院长。

美国工程院在美国科学院的授权下于 1964 年成立，是一个拥有大批杰出工程师的机构。它与美国科学院并列，拥有独立的行政权和人事权，与美国科学院一起担负为联邦政府提供咨询的责任。美国工程院倡导旨在满足国家需要的工程计划，鼓励教育和研究，表彰具有突出业绩的工程师。查尔斯·韦斯特博士是美国工程院院长。

医学院由美国科学院在 1970 年建立，旨在保证相关行业杰出专业人士对有关公共健康的政策事务的审查。根据国会宪章对美国科学院的授权，医学院为联邦政府提供咨询，同时自主地确定医疗、研究和教育方面的议题。哈维·芬伯格博士是医学院院长。

国家研究委员会由美国科学院在 1916 年组建，它负责科学院与科技界的联系，为科学院进一步获得知识及为联邦政府提供咨询的目标服务。委员会的职责依据科学院的总体政策来确定，已成为美国科学院和美国工程院的主要运行机构，为政府、公众、科学和工程界提供服务。委员会由科学院、工程院和医学院共同管理。拉尔夫・塞西隆博士和查尔斯・韦斯特博士分别是国家研究委员会的主席和副主席。

www.national-academies.org

致　谢

中美两国的官员和学术界的同行们为术语汇编编委会提供了很多想法和意见，他们经过讨论所形成的观点成为本术语汇编的重要基础。编委会在此对那些为术语汇编的全面性和准确性提供帮助的人士表示衷心的感谢。

本术语汇编还吸取了中美两国很多机构的现有成果。我们特别感谢核威胁倡议基金会(NTI)和蒙特雷国际研究所，让我们参考他们在 2002 年编写的核术语词典。我们还要感谢《国防名词大典——核能卷》编委会、《军备控制与裁军手册》编委会和《中国军事大百科》编委会，本术语汇编中许多术语和定义引自这些文献。

依照美国国家研究委员会的报告评审委员会以及中国原子能出版社和中国人民争取和平与裁军协会共同组成的联合评审委员会所授权的程序，来自不同领域的、持有不同观点的技术专家对术语汇编初稿进行了审查。独立评审的目的在于提出坦诚的批评性意见，使所出版的术语汇编能尽可能地完善，并达到客观、准确的标准。在评审期间，所提的意见和初稿都是保密的，以确保程序的独立和完整。我们在此感谢以下评审委员：

中方评审委员

钱绍钧　院士，中国人民解放军总装备部，研究员
吕　敏　院士，北京系统工程研究所，研究员
宋家树　院士，中国工程物理研究院，研究员
诸旭辉　中国核工业集团公司，研究员
严叔衡　中国核工业集团公司，研究员

刘恭梁　北京应用物理与计算数学研究所，研究员

牛　强　中国人民争取和平与裁军协会，秘书长

段占元　中国国防部，研究员

欧阳立平　中国现代国际关系研究院，研究员

卫广刚　原子能出版社，编辑

美方评审委员

Ping Lee　国家安全技术有限责任公司，部门负责人

Stephanie Lieggi　蒙特雷国际研究所，研究员

James Mulvenon　情报研究与分析中心，军工集团公司主任

Brad Roberts　国防分析研究所，研究员

Christopher Twomey　海军研究生院，助理教授，研究副主管

Jing-dong Yuan　蒙特雷国际研究所，东亚防扩散项目主任

尽管上述评审委员提供了很多有建设性的意见和建议，但是他们与术语汇编出版无关，也不会在出版前看到最终版本。在美国，术语汇编的评审工作受来自芝加哥大学的 R. Stephen Berry 的监督，他受国家科学院委托，负责确保依据既定程序对术语汇编进行独立审查，同时确保所有评审意见能够得到认真的考虑。相应地，在中国，评审工作受到钱绍钧院士的领导，他负责领导委员会对术语进行全面的检查和审核，特别是那些带定义的术语。编委会对术语汇编的最终内容，包括其客观性和准确性，全权负责。

前言

中国人民争取和平与裁军协会的中国科学家军备控制小组(CSGAC)和美国科学院国际安全和军备控制委员会(CISAC)已经交往了近二十年，双方共同讨论核军备控制、核不扩散、核能源和地区安全等问题，目标是在全球范围内尽量降低核武器使用的可能性和核扩散。

在丰富的交流活动中，在精通英汉双语的与会人员和翻译的帮助下，双方的讨论得以顺利进行。尽管 CSGAC 和 CISAC 长期以来相互了解，并且有许多共同的关切，但是将一种语言翻译成另一种语言绝非易事，常常会出现双方对某一术语产生不同解释的困境。

随着国际社会在不扩散核武器、反扩散和防止核恐怖主义方面的不断努力，同时随着核能应用和国际核查功能的日益扩展，母语分别是英文和中文的与会者就相关术语在两种语言中的定义取得共识是非常重要的。有的尽管不能达成共识，但重要的是要理解相关术语在对方语言中的用法，并且应意识到这些术语可能在对方语言中有着不同的甚至含糊不清的含义。

2006年4月，CSGAC和CISAC考虑共同编写一本非保密的核安全术语汇编，并且认为这一想法很有价值且切实可行。因此，双方组成了工作小组，共同拟定了术语汇编的框架结构，并由CSGAC提出了最初的版本。双方经过电子邮件频繁地交换意见，并于2006年9月和2007年3月在北京召开工作会，对术语汇编的框架和入选的条目进行细致深入的讨论。在此基础上，又通过电子邮件多次交换意见后，双方各自在本国组织权威专家小组对文本进行了审阅和评议，并把这些意见汇总在文本中，在2007年11月的双方工作会议上，CSGAC和CISAC对术语的条目、定义和参考文献等最终定稿。我们相信，这本由CSGAC和CISAC共同编写的术语汇编将成为政府部门、学术界和安全领域有价值的参考资料。

本汇编包含了大约 1 000 个术语，它旨在减少双方产生误解的可能性，消除在外交、合作、交流或其他活动进展过程中的障碍，因为其间准确无误的相互了解至关重要。这些术语分为三类。第一类只需要给出英汉对应的名词，而不需要定义。因为在我们讨论过程中，由一方对这些术语做出的定义很容易被另一方接受，不太可能引起误解。所以本汇编中大部分术语只有相互对应的中英文名称。

第二类是需要定义的术语，这些术语在一种语言中只有单一的定义，但在另一种语言中可能有几个定义，分别对应截然不同的几种情况。对于这些术语，我们会选用经讨论后确定的定义，并依次用两种语言呈现出来。

第三类是即使在同一种语言中也会有几种不同定义的术语，这些术语在不同的上下文中表示不同的对象、行动或概念。对于这类术语，虽然在很多情况下我们都同意其中对应的某个定义，但是我们还是认为有必要列出其在军事和外交等领域中可能出现的不同解释。

我们尽可能地从现有著作或汇编中选取术语的定义。优先考虑的是国际性文件，其次是政府官方文件，再次是一些有名望组织的出版物和一些重要文献，如美国科学院的出版物、中国出版的《军备控制与裁军手册》、《国防名词大典-核能卷》等。我们按照传统的汉英、英汉顺序将工作成果出版成册。此外，我们还以更“亲近”读者的格式制作了本汇编的网络版，网址是：http://www.cpapd.org.cn/webglossary和http://www8.nationalacademies.org/webglossary。

因为术语在不断变化，我们希望将来能出版本汇编的增补版；随着双方探讨范围的扩大，一些术语的定义将会变得更加清晰，我们将定期更新网络版。我们计划用一种透明的方式来做这些工作，使网络读者既能看到原先的版本，又能看到所做的修订。

编委会打算在本书出版大约一年后正式重审这些术语条目，并根据需要增补和修订。编委员欢迎您对本汇编提供保贵意见。我们的邮箱是：css@iapcm.ac.cn和cisac@nas.edu。

最后，我们特别感谢CSGAC的胡思得院士和CISAC的Richard Garwin博士在本汇编的整个编写过程中所提供的大量指导性意见。这两位著名科学家分别是中美编委会的领导人和词条编写的技术指导人，我们为他们的加入而深感自豪。

田东风　陆明世

田东风　　　　陆明世

2008 年 4 月

总 目

凡 例

一 编排

本术语汇编按汉语拼音字母顺序和英文单词字母顺序分两部分进行编排，分别称为中文部分和英文部分。每一部分的每一页都按相对应的中文和英文分为两栏，且中文部分的中文一栏在左，英文一栏在右；英文部分的英文一栏在左，中文一栏在右。

中文部分按汉语拼音字母排序。若词条中第一个汉字的拼音相同，则按阴平(即第一声，例：ā)、阳平(即第二声，例：á)、上声(即第三声，例：ǎ)和去声(即第四声，例：à)的声调顺序排序；同音、同调时，分别按汉字的笔画多少和笔顺排序。若第一个汉字的音、调、笔画和笔顺都相同，则按第二个汉字的音、调、笔画和笔顺排序，以下类推。

英文部分按英文单词字母顺序编排，字母不分大小写。

为便于读者按学科体系检索，本术语汇编正文之前列有全部条目的分类索引。第一级表示大类，第二级表示小类，第三级表示条目。条目之间不再分级。中文部分的类和条目仅以中文表示，跟在条目后面的数字表示该条目所在的页数；同样，英文部分的类和条目仅以英文表示，跟在条目后面的数字表示该条目所在的页数。例如：

核军备

核武器

战略核武器……………………………78

战术核武器……………………………78

二 条目内容

条目一般由条目名称、拼音、定义、出处、注、参见等内容组成。除条目名称和拼音是必有内容外，其他内容根据条目的需要而取舍；除拼音外，出现的各部分内容都有相对应的中、英文。

1 条目名称

条目名称通常是词或词组，且中文条目后面加注汉语拼音。例如：

核武器【héwǔqì】　　　　nuclear weapon

条目名称中出现圆括号( )时，圆括号内的内容或表示替代，或表示注解，或表示缩写。例如：

表示替代：地(水)下核爆炸

表示注解：杜皮克工艺(压水堆乏燃料直接用于坎杜反应堆的工艺)

表示缩写：指挥、控制、通信和情报系统(C3I 系统)

条目名称中出现符号“/”时，表示“/”前后的内容可通用。例如：

转用策略/转用途径

2 拼音

本术语汇编中汉语词条中的每个汉字依照普通话的语音系统，用汉语拼音字母注音，词与词的拼音之间以空格分隔。如：

战略核武器【zhànlüè héwǔqì】

轻声字则仅注音而不注声调。例如：

保障监督的质量保证 【bǎozhàng jiāndū de zhìliàng bǎozhèng】

条目名称中的非汉字部分，在汉语拼音中直接写非汉字符号。例如：

无源 γ 射线探测 【wúyuán γ shèxiàn tàncè】

条目名称中的标点符号在汉语拼音中省略。例如：

发方/收方差额 【fāfāng shōufāng chā’é】

3 定义及出处

条目定义的开始一般不重复条目名称。

本术语汇编对于词条定义的出处，一般只引述出现该定义的片段。如果引用的定义与原文一致，则在定义后面注明“源自:”；如果使用的定义在原文的基础上稍事修改，则在定义后面注明“改自:”。

个别词条如有两种或两种以上定义时，则分别列出定义内容及出处。

引用的定义都注明了参考文献序号及页数。参考文献详情可根据序号参阅书后的“参考文献”部分。

4 注

一个条目的内容需要补充注释时，采用“注”的方式。例如：

标签【biāoqiān】

……

注：有源标签工作时需要电源，但无源标签不需要电源。

5 参见

一个条目的内容涉及其他条目时，采用“参见”的方式。例如：

原子弹弹芯【yuánzǐdàn dànxīn】

参见“弹芯”

三 参考文献

本部分包含了术语汇编中引用文献的详细信息。参考文献分别用中文和英文列出，中英文格式统一，以便于理解，并提供尽量多的信息，以便于读者找到原文献。参考文献的信息一般按以下顺序排列：作者、篇名、出版地、出版社、出版日期、网上可查阅的最近日期和网址等信息。有些参考文献还包含了版本、卷号或文件号等信息。由于有些参考文献被多次引用，术语汇编正文的定义部分也列出了该定义在参考文献中的页码。

四 其他

本术语汇编所用汉字，以中国国家语言文字工作委员会 1986 年 10 月重新发表的《简化字总表》为准。本术语汇编所用的中文标点符号，以《中华人民共和国国家标准》GB/T 15834—1995 为准。本术语汇编所用的数字，以《中华人民共和国国家标准》GB/T 15835—1995 为准，但未进行数字分节。本术语汇编所用的中文计量单位和科学技术符号，以《中华人民共和国国家标准》GB 3100～3102—93 为准。数字除习惯用汉字表示的外，一般采用阿拉伯数字。

索 引

(按汉语拼音次序)

一 军备控制与裁军

1 军备控制、裁军与国际安全

2 军备控制和裁军的国际法

3 日内瓦和联合国主要裁军机构

4 核军备控制与裁军的条约、协定

索
引

二 核军备

1 核战略

2 核武器

3 核武器运载与发射系统

三 禁止核试验

1 禁止核试验的条约

2 核试验与监测

四 禁止生产核武器用的裂变材料

1 与国际原子能机构保障监督有关的法律文书及文件

索引

2 国际原子能机构保障监督

3 核材料和非核材料

4 核及核有关活动与装置

5 核材料衡算

6 核材料核查与监测

五 不扩散

六 建立信任措施

七 军备控制与裁军条约的核查

八 核科学基础

γ辐射监测和能谱分析 【γ fúshè jiāncè hé néngpǔ fēnxī】	**gamma radiation monitoring and energy spectrum analysis**
INFCIRC/153 型保障监督协定 **(IAEA)** 【INFCIRC 153 xíng bǎozhàng jiāndū xiédìng】	**INFCIRC/153 safeguards agreement (IAEA)**
INFCIRC/66 型保障监督协定 **(IAEA)** 【INFCIRC 66 xíng bǎozhàng jiāndū xiédìng】	**INFCIRC/66 safeguards agreement (IAEA)**
X 射线辐照引起的力学损伤 【X shèxiàn fúzhào yǐnqǐ de lìxué sǔnshāng】	**mechanical damage induced by X-ray irradiation**
八国集团"防止大规模杀伤性武器和材料扩散的全球伙伴计划" 【bāguó jítuán fángzhǐ dàguīmó shāshāngxìng wǔqì hé cáiliào kuòsàn de quánqiú huǒbàn jìhuà】 该计划是八国集团(俄罗斯、美国、英国、法国、日本、德国、加拿大和意大利)于 2002 年提出的，旨在通过与裁军、不扩散、反恐和核安全有关的项目，防止大规模杀伤性武器扩散到恐怖主义者或其支持者手中。最初目标是在俄罗斯开展为期 10 年耗资 200 亿美元的项目，现八国集团全球伙伴关系已经扩展到八国以外的国家。(改自：参考文献[42-43])	**G-8 Global Partnership Against the Spread of Weapons and Materials of Mass Destruction** Launched in 2002 by the G 8 (Russian, the U.S., Britian, France, Japan, Germany, Canada and Italy), this effort aims to prevent the proliferation of weapons of mass destruction to terrorists or those who support them through projects pertaining to disarmament, nonproliferation, counterterrorism and nuclear safety. Originally targeted at carrying out $20 billion of projects in Russia over 10 years, the G-8 Global Partnership has expanded to include additional countries. (Modified from: References [42-43])
霸权主义【bàquánzhǔyì】	**hegemonism**
半衰期【bànshuāiqī】	**half-life**
保护区实体屏障 【bǎohùqū shítǐ píngzhàng】	**physical barrier for protected sections**
保护系统完整性 【bǎohù xìtǒng wánzhěngxìng】	**integrity of protection system**

保障监督标准 【bǎozhàng jiāndū biāozhǔn】	**safeguards criteria**
保障监督的质量保证 【bǎozhàng jiāndū de zhìliàng bǎozhèng】 在国际原子能机构保障监督体系下，确保对所有会影响保障监督实施质量的活动进行系统化监控的一种管理手段。(源自：参考文献[4]，3.36)	**safeguards quality assurance** In the context of IAEA safeguards, a management tool for ensuring a systematic approach to all of the activities affecting the quality of the safeguards implementation. (From: Reference [4], 3.36)
保障监督结论 【bǎozhàng jiāndū jiélùn】	**safeguards conclusion**
保障监督协定 【bǎozhàng jiāndū xiédìng】	**Safeguards Agreement**
爆心投影点【bàoxīn tóuyǐngdiǎn】	**ground zero**
备忘录【bèiwànglù】	**memorandum**
备用弹头【bèiyòng dàntóu】	**spare warhead**
备用性核武库【bèiyòngxìng héwǔkù】 美国现役核武库的一部分，作为响应力量的一部分予以保留，用来加强作战部署的力量以应对潜在的意外事故、突发的事件或显现的威胁。(改自：参考文献[66] p4，[67-68])	**hedge warheads stockpile** One part of the U.S. active stockpile of warheads, retained as part of the responsive force, to be used to augment the operationally deployed force in order to meet potential contingencies, unanticipated events or emerging threats. (Modified from: Reference [66], p4; [67-68])
比等效百万吨数 【bǐděngxiào bǎiwàndūnshù】	**equivalent megatonnage-to-weight ratio**
比例爆高【bǐlì bàogāo】	**scaled height of burst**
比例爆深【bǐlì bàoshēn】	**scaled depth of burst**
比威力【bǐwēilì】	**yield-to-weight ratio**
闭式核燃料循环 【bìshì héránliào xúnhuán】 核燃料循环通常有两种类型。一种	**closed nuclear fuel cycle** There are two common types of nuclear fuel cycle. One is the “open” fuel cycle,

是“开式”燃料循环，即乏燃料不经过后处理，在最终处置前以废料形式储存。另一种是“闭式”燃料循环，即乏燃料经过后处理从裂变产物中分离出铀和钚。铀和钚都可作为新的燃料元件循环使用。(源自：参考文献[14]，p1-2)	in which the spent fuel is not reprocessed but kept in storage pending eventual disposal as waste. The other is the “closed” fuel cycle, where the spent fuel is reprocessed and the uranium and plutonium separated from the fission products. Both the uranium and the plutonium can be recycled into new fuel elements. (From: Reference [14], p1-2)
变换打击目标能力【biànhuàn dǎjī mùbiāo nénglì】	**target-changing capability**
标签【biāoqiān】 在军备控制条约的限制对象上，为便于核查而设置的某种独特标志。标签必须具有固有的特征，不能复制、转移、篡改或探测，同时要稳定、可靠、便宜。(源自：参考文献[1]，p496) 注：有源标签工作时需要电源，但无源标签不需要电源。	**tag** A unique identifier set up for facilitating verification of items restricted by arms control treaties. A tag must have intrinsic characteristic which make it difficult to be duplicated, transferred, tampered or detected. A tag should also be stable, credible and inexpensive. (From: Reference [1], p496) Note: An active tag requires electrical power, while a passive tag works without a power supply.
标识数据【biāoshí shùjù】	**identity (identification) data**
标准事件筛选判据【biāozhǔn shìjiàn shāixuǎn pànjù】	**standard event screening criteria**
玻璃固化【bōli gùhuà】	**glass solidification**
不结盟运动【bùjiéméng yùndòng】	**nonaligned movement**
不扩散【bùkuòsàn】	**non-proliferation**
不扩散核武器条约【bùkuòsàn héwǔqì tiáoyuē】	**Treaty on the Non-Proliferation of Nuclear Weapons (NPT)**
《不扩散核武器条约》审议会【bùkuòsàn héwǔqì tiáoyuē shěnyìhuì】	**NPT Review Conferences**

不明材料量【bùmíng cáiliàoliàng】	**material unaccounted for (MUF)**
不实施国际原子能机构的保障监督【bùshíshī guójì yuánzǐnéng jīgòu de bǎozhàng jiāndū】	**non-application of IAEA safeguards**
不首先使用核武器【bù shǒuxiān shǐyòng héwǔqì】	**no-first-use of nuclear weapons**
不停堆换料动力堆【bùtíngduī huànliào dònglìduī】	**on-load refuelled power reactor**
不通知视察【bùtōngzhī shìchá】	**unannounced inspection**
不遵约【bùzūnyuē】	**non-compliance**
钚【bù】	**plutonium**
钚管理指导原则【bù guǎnlǐ zhǐdǎo yuánzé】 该指导原则由五个核武器国家和德国、日本、比利时、瑞士等九国于1997年通过，它着眼于按照国际约定(包括它们在NPT下的义务，欧共体成员国还有欧洲原子能联营条约下的义务)和IAEA的保障监督协定确保对持有的钚进行安全有效的管理。该指导原则描述了在接受该指导原则下适用于钚的核材料衡算体制、实体保护措施和国际运输手续。它还进一步指定了参与国要发布的有关钚管理的信息，包括他们所持有的民用未辐照钚和民用反应堆乏燃料中含有的钚估量的年度申报。(源自：参考文献[1]，p409；[4]，1.30)	**Guidelines for the Management of Plutonium** The Guidelines adopted by nine states (the five nuclear weapon states and Germany, Japan, Belgium and Switzerland) in 1997, with a view to ensuring that holdings of plutonium are managed safely and effectively in accordance with international commitments, including their obligations under the NPT (and, for states that are members of the European Community, also under the Euratom Treaty), and with their safeguards agreements with the IAEA. The Guidelines describe, inter alia, the nuclear material accountancy system, physical protection measures and international transfer procedures applicable to the plutonium subject to the Guidelines. They further specify the information to be published by the participating States in respect of plutonium management, including

	annual statements of their holdings of civil unirradiated plutonium and of their estimates of plutonium contained in spent civil reactor fuel. (From: Reference [1], p409；[4], 1.30)
钚合金【bùhéjīn】	**plutonium alloy**
钚净化循环【bù jìnghuà xúnhuán】	**plutonium decontamination cycle**
钚再循环【bù zàixúnhuán】 将从乏燃料中回收得到的钚在反应堆内再使用的过程。(源自：参考文献[2]，p22) 注：在 DUPIC 过程中，轻水堆的乏燃料棒只需机械处理而不需化学后处理即可直接作为 CANDU 型重水动力堆的燃料。(源自：参考文献[32]，p25-40)	**plutonium recycling** A process of reusing in nuclear reactors the plutonium extracted from spent fuel. (From: Reference [2], p22) Note: In the DUPIC process, spent LWR fuel rods are directly used as fuel for CANDU-type heavy-water power reactors, with only mechanical modifications and not chemical reprocessing. (From: Reference [32], p25-40)
部署弹头的检修 【bùshǔ dàntóu de jiǎnxiū】	**examine and repair deployed warhead**
擦拭取样【cāshì qǔyàng】 一种环境样品的收集方法，它通过用一块超洁净介质(例如布)擦拭物体表面以获取物体表面残留的材料痕迹。(源自：参考文献[4]，9.4)	**swipe sampling** The collection of environmental samples by swiping a surface with a piece of ultraclean medium (such as cloth) to remove from the surface traces of the materials present. (From: Reference [4], 9.4)
材料类别【cáiliào lèibié】	**material category**
材料类型【cáiliào lèixíng】	**material type**
材料平衡区的账面存量 【cáiliào pínghéngqū de zhàngmiàn cúnliàng】	**book inventory of a material balance area**

材料平衡周期 【cáiliào pínghéng zhōuqī】	**material balance period (MBP)**
材料说明【cáiliào shuōmíng】	**material description**
材料形态【cáiliào xíngtài】	**material form**
裁军【cáijūn】	**disarmament**
裁军谈判会议 【cáijūn tánpàn huìyì】	**Conference on Disarmament (CD)**
裁军谈判会议特设委员会【cáijūn tánpàn huìyì tèshè wěiyuánhuì】	**Ad Hoc Committee of Conference on Disarmament**
裁军谈判委员会 【cáijūn tánpàn wěiyuánhuì】	**Committee on Disarmament**
裁军委员会会议 【cáijūn wěiyuánhuì huìyì】	**Conference of the Committee on Disarmament (CCD)**
采办策略/采办途径 【cǎibàn cèlüè cǎibàn tújìng】 某国谋取用于制造核爆炸装置的核材料的一种(设想)策略。(源自：参考文献[4]，3.8)	**acquisition strategy/acquisition path** A (hypothetical) scheme which a State could consider to acquire nuclear material usable for manufacturing a nuclear explosive device. (From: Reference [4], 3.8)
参考物质【cānkǎo wùzhì】	**reference material**
产氚堆【chǎn chuān duī】	**tritium production reactor**
产氚方法【chǎnchuān fāngfǎ】	**methods of tritium production**
超临界气体离心机 【chāolínjiè qìtǐ líxīnjī】	**supercritical gas centrifuge**
超越遏制战略 【chāoyuè èzhì zhànlüè】	**strategy of going beyond containment**
成像侦察卫星 【chéngxiàng zhēnchá wèixīng】	**imaging reconnaissance satellite**
冲击波弹【chōngjībō dàn】	**shock wave weapon**
冲击波毁伤效应 【chōngjībō huǐshāng xiàoyìng】	**damaging and injuring effects of shock wave**
冲击载荷【chōngjī zàihè】	**shock wave load**

重访周期 【chóngfǎng zhōuqī】	**revisit period**
重新瞄准能力 【chóngxīn miáozhǔn nénglì】	**retargeting capability**
出入口控制 【chūrùkǒu kòngzhì】	**entrance and exit control**
初始视察【chūshǐ shìchá】	**initial inspection**
触发清单【chùfā qīngdān】 核供应国集团规定，向无核武器国家出口“清单”上的项目，要“触发”国际原子能机构的保障监督。(源自：参考文献[1]，p407)	**trigger list** The NSG prescribes that items on the list exported to non-nuclear-weapon states should trigger the IAEA safe-guards. (From: Reference [1], p407)
氚【chuān】	**tritium**
次临界安全模拟实验系统 【cìlínjiè ānquán mónǐ shíyàn xìtǒng】	**subcritical safety simulation experiment system**
次临界度【cìlínjiè dù】	**subcriticality**
次临界实验【cìlínjiè shíyàn】 实验中裂变系统处于次临界状态的爆轰流体动力学实验，裂变材料的用量以不会发生自持链式裂变核反应为限。(改自:参考文献[1]，p214)	**subcritical experiment** Hydrodynamic detonation experiment in which the fission system remains subcritical, the material used would not exceed the amount that may produce a self-sustaining chain reaction. (Modified from: Reference [1], p214)
次临界装置【cìlínjiè zhuāngzhì】	**subcritical assembly**
次声监测【cìshēng jiāncè】	**infrasound monitoring**
存量【cúnliàng】	**inventory**
存量变化【cúnliàng biànhuà】	**inventory change**
存留废物【cúnliú fèiwù】	**retained waste**
打击核恐怖主义全球行动倡议 【dǎjī hékǒngbùzhǔyì quánqiú xíngdòng chàngyì】 2006 年由美国和俄国发起，旨在防止恐怖主义分子获取核材料的倡	**Global Initiative to Combat Nuclear Terrorism** Launched in 2006 by the United States and Russia, the initiative aims to prevent terrorist access to nuclear

议，具体措施包括：改善核及放射性材料的衡算与安全，加强对民用核设施的保护，提高对核及放射性物质探测能力以防止非法走私。(源自：参考文献[44])	materials by improving accounting and security of radioactive and nuclear materials, enhancing security at civilian nuclear facilities, and improving detection of nuclear and radioactive materials to prevent illicit trafficking. (From: Reference [44])
打击军事力量【dǎjī jūnshì lìliàng】 在任何可引发冲突的情况下，使用战略空军和导弹力量摧毁或使选定的敌方军事力量失效。(源自：参考文献[9]，p128)	**counterforce strike** The employment of strategic air and missile forces in an effort to destroy, or render impotent, selected military capabilities of an enemy force under any of the circumstances by which hostilities may be initiated. (From: Reference [9], p128)
打击社会财富【dǎjī shèhuì cáifù】 打击敌方有价值的非军事目标，如人口和工业设施。(改自：参考文献[27])	**countervalue strike** Striking non-military assets of value to the enemy, such as population and industry centers. (Modified from: Reference [27])
大规模报复战略【dàguīmó bàofù zhànlüè】	**strategy of massive retaliation**
大国协调【dàguó xiétiáo】	**concert of powers**
大陆架【dàlùjià】	**continental shelf**
大气层核爆炸取样技术【dàqìcéng hébàozhà qǔyàng jìshù】	**sampling technology of atmospheric nuclear explosion**
大气层核试验【dàqìcéng héshìyàn】	**atmospheric nuclear test**
大气层核试验的安全问题【dàqìcéng héshìyàn de ānquán wèntí】	**safety problems of atmospheric nuclear test**
代表性样品【dàibiǎoxìng yàngpǐn】	**representative sample**
单位分离功能耗【dānwèi fēnlígōng nénghào】	**energy consumption of unit separative work**
单循环流程【dānxúnhuán liúchéng】	**single-cycle process**
弹道导弹潜艇【dàndàodǎodàn qiántǐng】	**ballistic-missile submarine**

弹道导弹预警系统 【dàndàodǎodàn yùjǐng xìtǒng】	**ballistic-missile early warning system**
弹芯【dànxīn】 安置在内爆装置中心、通常有铍或其他金属包层的核炸药材料球体或壳体。(改自：参考文献[11]，p90)	**pit** The sphere or shell of nuclear explosive material at the center of an implosion device, usually clad with beryllium or another metal. (Modified from: Reference [11], p90)
当量剂量【dāngliàng jìliàng】	**equivalent dose**
氘【dāo】	**deuterium**
氘氚化锂【dāochuānhuàlǐ】	**lithium deutero-tritide**
氘化锂【dāohuàlǐ】	**lithium deuteride**
导弹技术控制制度 【dǎodàn jìshù kòngzhì zhìdù】 美国等西方国家 1987 年制定的，旨在防止用于运载大规模杀伤性武器的投掷系统(有人驾驶飞机除外)及有关设备和技术扩散的控制制度。该制度由“准则”和“设备与技术附件“两个文件组成，把限制项目(导弹、分系统、部件，生产设施和有关技术)分成两大类。第一类项目为“最敏感项目”，一般不得转让。第二类项目为军民两用项目，出口时要以许可证方式逐件审批，保证不用于包含第一类项目的系统。1993 年成员国对“准则”进行了修改，把原版中控制“核武器运载系统”的转让改成控制“大规模杀伤性武器(即核、生、化武器)运载系统”的转让。截至 2007 年底，该制	**Missile Technology Control Regime (MTCR)** The MTCR was originally established in 1987 by western countries. It is a regime that aims to restrict the proliferation of systems (except manned air vehicles), equipments and technologies intended for the delivery of weapons of mass destruction (WMD). The MTCR includes the Guidelines and the Equipment and Technology Annex, and it divides controlled items (missiles along with their subsystems and components, production equipments and related technologies) into two category. Category I items are the most sensitive items, commonly the transfer of them will not be authorized. Category II items are dual-use items, which should be examined and approved case-by-case subject to export license, and be guaranteed not to be used in projects including Category I items. In 1993, member states modified the Guidelines. “Control the transfer of

度有 34 个成员国。(改自：参考文献[1]，p410)	nuclear weapons delivery systems", in the original version was modified to "control the transfer of weapons of mass destruction (nuclear, biological, chemical weapon) delivery systems". Up to the end of 2007, the Regime has 34 member states. (Modified from: Reference [1], p410)
导弹精度【dǎodàn jīngdù】	**missile accuracy**
导弹遥测信号【dǎodàn yáocè xìnhào】	**telemetry signal for missiles**
等效百万吨数【děngxiào báiwàndūnshù】 以百万吨 TNT 当量为单位计量核弹威力的数值的三分之二次方。用公式可表示为 $EMT=(Y/Y_0)^{2/3}$。式中 Y 为核弹威力，Y_0 为一百万吨 TNT 当量。(改自：参考文献[3]，p115-116)	**equivalent megatonnage** The 2/3 power of the yield of a nuclear warhead measured by megaton TNT equivalent. The formula is $EMT=(Y/Y_0)^{2/3}$, where Y is the yield of a nuclear warhead and Y_0 is one megaton TNT equivalent. (Modified from: Reference [3], p115-116)
低放废物【dīfàng fèiwù】	**low level radioactive waste**
低浓铀【dīnóngyóu】	**low-enriched uranium (LEU)**
低强度冲突理论【dīqiángdù chōngtū lǐlùn】	**theory of low intensity conflict**
地面分辨率/空间分辨率【dìmiàn fēnbiànlǜ kōngjiān fēnbiànlǜ】	**ground resolution/spatial resolution**
地面或地下核爆炸毁伤效应【dìmiàn huò dìxià hébàozhà huǐshāng xiàoyìng】	**damaging and injuring effects of surface or underground nuclear explosion**
地区核材料衡算和控制系统【dìqū hécáiliào héngsuàn hé kòngzhì xìtǒng】	**regional system of accounting for and control of nuclear material (RSAC)**
地(水)面核爆炸【dìshuǐmiàn hébàozhà】	**nuclear land (water) surface burst**
地(水)下核爆炸【dìshuǐxià hébàozhà】	**nuclear underground (or underwater) burst**

地下发射井【dìxià fāshèjǐng】	**silo**
地下核爆炸取样技术 【dìxià hébàozhà qǔyàng jìshù】	**sampling technology of underground nuclear explosion**
地下核试验【dìxià héshìyàn】	**underground nuclear test**
地下核试验的安全问题 【dìxià héshìyàn de ānquán wèntí】	**safety problems of underground nuclear test**
地下井冷发射【dìxiàjǐng lěngfāshè】	**silo cold launch**
地下井热发射【dìxiàjǐng rèfāshè】	**silo hot launch**
地震监测【dìzhèn jiāncè】	**seismic monitoring**
地震监测系统【dìzhèn jiāncè xìtǒng】	**seismic monitoring system**
地质处置库【dìzhì chǔzhìkù】	**geological repository**
第二次核打击【dì' èrcì hédǎjī】 对敌方第一次核袭击的报复性核打击。(改自：参考文献[2]，p62)	**nuclear second strike** Retaliatory nuclear attack following an enemy's first nuclear attack. (Modified from: Reference [2], p62)
第二代核武器【dì'èrdài héwǔqì】	**second-generation nuclear weapon**
第三代核武器【dìsāndài héwǔqì】	**third-generation nuclear weapon**
第一次核打击【dìyīcì hédǎjī】 1 在对手能够使用任何战略武器之前率先发动核攻击。首次打击是给对手造成极大的破坏致使其失去发起有效反击能力的核进攻。(源自：参考文献[6]，p72) 2 对敌方战略核力量的首次打击。这种打击可用于试图摧毁敌方的报复(第二次打击)能力。(源自：参考文献[8])	**nuclear first strike** 1 The launching of an initial nuclear attack before one's opponent is able to use any strategic weapon. First strike is a nuclear attack carried out at such a devastatingly high level of destruction as to nullify an enemy's capability to launch a major counterstrike. (From: Reference [6], p72) 2 An initial attack on an opponent's strategic nuclear forces. Such an attack may be undertaken in an attempt to destroy an enemy's retaliatory (second-strike) capability. (From: Reference [8])

第一代核武器【dìyīdài héwǔqì】	**first-generation nuclear weapon**
点目标【diǎn mùbiāo】	**point target**
点样品【diǎn yàngpǐn】 在一个特定地区环境为确定能够在接近泄漏点临近地区发现泄漏物质的源的特征而采集的样品。(源自：参考文献[4]，9.5)	**point sample** An environmental sample taken in one particular area to characterize one source of released material which can be found in a contiguous area adjacent to a release point. (From: Reference [4], 9.5)
电磁脉冲弹【diàncí màichōng dàn】 一种设计成能加强核武器电磁脉冲效应的核爆炸装置。(源自：参考文献[20])	**electromagnetic pulse weapon** A nuclear explosive designed to enhance the electromagnetic pulse radiated by a nuclear weapon. (From: Reference [20])
电子【diànzǐ】	**electron**
电子枪【diànzǐqiāng】	**electron gun**
电子系统的瞬态辐射效应【diànzǐ xìtǒng de shùntài fúshè xiàoyìng】	**transient radiation effects on electronics**
电子系统的永久性辐射损伤【diànzǐ xìtǒng de yǒngjiǔxìng fúshè sǔnshāng】	**permanent radiation damage in electronics**
电子侦察卫星【diànzǐ zhēnchá wèixīng】	**electronic reconnaissance satellite/electronic intelligence (ELINT) satellite**
东盟地区论坛【dōngméng dìqū lùntán】	**ASEAN (Association of Southeast Asian Nations) Regional Forum**
东南亚无核武器区条约(曼谷条约)【dōngnányà wúhéwǔqìqū tiáoyuē màngǔ tiáoyuē】	**Treaty on the Southeast Asia Nuclear Weapon-Free Zone (Treaty of Bangkok)**
动力堆【dònglìduī】	**power reactor**
冻结【dòngjié】	**freeze**

杜皮克工艺【dùpíkè gōngyì】 (压水堆乏燃料直接用于坎杜反应堆的工艺)	**DUPIC (Direct Use of Spent PWR fuel in CANDU reactors) process**
对照样品【duìzhào yàngpǐn】	**control sample**
钝感高能炸药 【dùngǎn gāonéng zhàyào】	**insensitive high explosive**
多层分离膜/复合分离膜 【duōcéng fēnlímó fùhé fēnlímó】 由多层不同结构的多孔膜紧密叠合组成的分离膜。(源自：参考文献[2]，p81)	**complex (diffusion) barrier** A kind of (isotope) separation barrier composed of multiple layers of compactly overlapped porous barriers with different structure. (From: Reference [2], p81)
多裂变体次临界安全实验 【duōlièbiàntǐ cìlínjiè ānquán shíyàn】	**multi-fissile body subcritical safety experiment**
遏制战略【èzhì zhànlüè】 美国在冷战初期试图阻止苏联的扩张和防止一些国家在政治上走向苏联领导的共产主义的外交政策战略。(改自：参考文献[40])	**containment strategy** Refers to the foreign policy strategy of the United States during the Cold War in which it attempted to stop the expansion of the Soviet Union and to prevent nations moving politically towards communism led by the Soviet Union. (Modified from: Reference [40])
遏制转用【èzhì zhuǎnyòng】	**deterrence of diversion**
21 国集团【èrshíyīguó jítuán】	**Group of 21**
二氧化钚【èryǎnghuàbù】	**plutonium dioxide**
二氧化铀【èryǎnghuàyóu】	**uranium dioxide**
发方/收方差额 【fāfāng shōufāng chā'é】	**shipper/receiver difference (SRD)**
乏燃料【fáránliào】	**spent fuel**
乏燃料的冷却 【fáránliào de lěngquè】	**cooling of spent fuel**
乏燃料管理安全和放射性废物管理安全联合公约 【fáránliào guǎnlǐ ānquán hé fàngshè	**Spent Fuel Management Safety and Radioactive Waste Management Safety Joint**

xìng fèiwù guǎnlǐ ānquán liánhé gōngyuē】	**Convention**
乏燃料贮存【fáránliào zhùcún】	**spent fuel storage**
反弹道导弹的导弹【fǎndàndàodǎodàn de dǎodàn】	**anti-ballistic-missile missile**
反胁迫报警【fǎnxiépò bàojǐng】 又称反劫持报警。给值班、巡逻人员配备的隐蔽报警装置。(改自：参考文献[2]，p91)	**anti-coercion alarm** Also called anti-hijack alarm. The concealed warning device provided for guards on duty or on patrol. (Modified from: Reference [2], p91)
反应堆【fǎnyìngduī】	**reactor**
反应堆分类【fǎnyìngduī fēnlèi】	**classification of reactor**
反应堆级钚【fǎnyìngduījí bù】 通常指钚-240 含量大于 18%的钚。(改自：参考文献[2]，p93)	**reactor-grade plutonium** Plutonium containing more than 18% Pu-240. (Modified from: Reference [2], p93)
方差 σ^2【fāngchā σ^2】	**variance σ^2**
防御性战略【fángyùxìng zhànlüè】 在全局上采取承受、逐步削弱和阻止的态势，防备和抗击敌人的进攻。(改自：参考文献[18]，p36-37)	**defensive strategy** To guard against and resist the enemy's attack by means of a strategy based on operations that absorb, progressively weaken and block such an attack. (Modified from: Reference [18], p36-37)
放射性沉降【fàngshèxìng chénjiàng】	**radioactive fallout**
放射性废物【fàngshèxìng fèiwù】	**radioactive waste**
放射性废物处置【fàngshèxìng fèiwù chǔzhì】	**radioactive waste disposal**
放射性废液处理【fàngshèxìng fèiyè chǔlǐ】	**processing of radioactive liquid waste**
放射性固体废物处理【fàngshèxìng gùtǐ fèiwù chǔlǐ】	**treatment of radioactive solid waste**

放射性核素监测 【fàngshèxìng hésù jiāncè】 通过收集、分析、测量各种放射性核素，以达到监测相关核活动目的的方法。(改自：参考文献[1]，p486)	**radionuclide monitoring** A method for monitoring nuclear related activity through collecting, analyzing, and measuring different kinds of radionuclides. (Modified from: Reference [1], p486)
放射性活度【fàngshèxìng huódù】	**radioactivity**
放射性气体取样与探测 【fàngshèxìng qìtǐ qǔyàng yǔ tàncè】	**radioactive gas sampling and detecting**
放射性同位素 【fàngshèxìng tóngwèisù】	**radioisotope**
放射性物质散布装置【fàngshèxìng wùzhì sànbù zhuāngzhì】 参见“脏弹”	**radiological dispersal device (RDD)** Refer to **“dirty bomb”**
放射性烟云【fàngshèxìng yānyún】	**radioactive cloud**
放射性沾染【fàngshèxìng zhānrǎn】	**radioactive contamination**
放射性沾染效应 【fàngshèxìng zhānrǎn xiàoyìng】	**effects of radioactive contamination**
非对称战争【fēiduìchèn zhànzhēng】 任何一方使用了不同的武器、战术或战略的战争。“所有战略都基于非对称性原则进行谋划和实施，因此理性运筹的战争都具有非对称性特征。”(源自：参考文献[55]，p102-108)	**asymmetric warfare** A war in which either side employs a different weapon, tactic or strategy. “All strategy works on asymmetries, so asymmetric warfare is representative of all rationally executed warfare.” (From: Reference [55], p102-108)
非核重型轰炸机基线展示 【fēihé zhòngxíng hōngzhàjī jīxiàn zhǎnshì】	**baseline exhibition for non-nuclear heavy bombers**
非现役弹头【fēi xiànyì dàntóu】	**inactive warhead**
非现役核武库【fēi xiànyì héwǔkù】	**inactive nuclear stockpile**
非直接使用材料 【fēi zhíjiē shǐyòng cáiliào】 除直接使用材料以外的所有核材料。它包括：贫化铀、天然铀和低	**indirect use material** All nuclear material except direct use material. It includes: depleted, natural and low enriched uranium, and thorium,

浓缩铀以及钚，所有这些材料都必须经过进一步加工以生产直接使用材料。(源自：参考文献[4]，4.26)	all of which must be further processed in order to produce direct use material. (From: Reference [4], 4.26)
废物固化【fèiwù gùhuà】	**waste solidification**
废物贮存【fèiwù zhùcún】	**waste storage**
沸水堆【fèishuǐduī】	**boiling water reactor (BWR)**
分导式多弹头【fēndǎoshì duōdàntóu】	**multiple independently targetable reentry vehicle (MIRV)**
分离单元【fēnlí dānyuán】	**separative element**
分离功【fēnlígōng】 把一定量的铀浓缩到一定的铀-235丰度所需要投入的工作量，表达为千克分离功单位(kgSWU)或吨分离功单位(tSWU)。(源自：参考文献[26]，p213)	**separative work** The required work to enrich uranium to a certain level of U-235 concentration. It is described in terms of kg Separative Work Unit (kgSWU) or ton Separative Work Unit (tSWU). (From：Reference [26], p213)
分离功单位【fēnlígōng dānwèi】	**separative work unit**
分离功率【fēnlí gōnglǜ】 一个分离单元或一个分离级联在单位时间所能提供的分离功。(改自：参考文献[2]，p125)	**separative power** A unit for measuring separative work per unit time provided by a separating unit or a separating cascade. (Modified from: Reference [2], p125)
分离级【fēnlíjí】	**separation stage**
分离膜【fēnlímó】	**diffusion barrier**
分离膜的渗透性 【fēnlímó de shèntòuxìng】	**permeability of barrier**
分离膜效率【fēnlímó xiàolǜ】 分离膜的实际浓缩因子与理想浓缩因子的比值。由于非纯分子流和膜后反扩散的影响，分离膜的实际浓缩因子通常小于理想浓缩因子。(改	**efficiency of barrier** The ratio of a porous barrier's real enrichment factor to its theoretical maximum enrichment factor. Because of non-ideal molecular flow and back diffusion, the real enrichment factor is less than the theoretical maximum

自：参考文献[2]，p126)	enrichment factor. (Modified from: Reference [2], p126)
分子流【fēnzǐliú】	**molecular flow**
封记【fēngjì】 用以紧紧地或完全地封闭或保护某物，俗称封条或封签。利用做特殊标记的方法在被核查设备或部件加封条，以防止武器及武器部件被转移和改动的措施。封记必须具有防止篡改和防伪造的特性，具有唯一性，不能复制，有很强的置信度，同时又要保证被核查设备或部件不受影响或不被改变，不揭示被核查设施的敏感信息。应用中的封记有光纤封记、焊缝封记、电子封记和超声封记等。(源自：参考文献[1]，p496) 注：有源封记工作时需要电源，但无源封记不需要电源。	**seal** Anything that tightly or completely closes or secures a thing. A seal with special markers is usually applied to those inspected equipments or components in order to prevent weapons and related components from being transferred and modified. A seal must be tamper-proof and counterfeit-proof and it must be unique and hard to duplicate with high confidence. It also should guarantee that inspected equipments or components remain unaffected or unchanged and that sensitive information related to the inspected facilities would not be revealed. Seals currently in application include fiber seal, welding seal, electric seal and ultrasonic seal etc. (From: Reference [1], p496) Note: An active seal requires electrical power, while a passive seal works without a power supply.
氟化挥发法【fúhuà huīfāfǎ】	**fluoride volatility process**
辐射【fúshè】	**radiation**
辐射波型电磁脉冲模拟器 【fúshèbōxíng diàncí màichōng mónǐqì】	**electromagnetic-pulse radiation-wave type simulator**
辐射加固的电子器件 【fúshè jiāgù de diànzǐ qìjiàn】	**radiation-hardened electronic components**
附加议定书【fùjiā yìdìngshū】	**Additional Protocol**
干法后处理【gānfǎ hòuchǔlǐ】	**dry reprocessing**
干法贮存【gānfǎ zhùcún】	**dry storage**

干净氢弹【gānjìng qīngdàn】	**clean hydrogen bomb**
干扰【gānrǎo】	**tampering**
感生放射性弹【gǎnshēng fàngshèxìngdàn】 利用核爆中子感生的放射性同位素增大放射性沾染的一种氢弹。1950年2月匈牙利物理学家L•西拉德最早提出这种弹的设想—"钴弹"。但并没有人制造和试验。(源自：参考文献[2]，p63)	**induced-radioactivity bomb** A type of hydrogen bomb that utilizes radioisotopes induced by neutrons during a nuclear explosion to increase radioactive contamination. In February 1950 Hungarian physicist Leo Szilard published the concept of this bomb — the "cobalt bomb". However no state manufactures and tests this kind of bomb. (From: Reference [2], p63)
高放废物【gāofàngfèiwù】	**high level radioactive waste**
高分辨率灵敏照相机【gāofēnbiànlǜ língmǐn zhàoxiàngjī】	**high resolution sensing camera**
高技术战争【gāojìshù zhànzhēng】	**high-technology warfare**
高空核爆炸【gāokōng hébàozhà】	**nuclear high altitude burst**
高空核爆炸电磁脉冲【gāokōng hébàozhà diàncí màichōng】	**electromagnetic pulse of high-altitude nuclear explosion**
高浓铀【gāonóngyóu】	**high-enriched uranium (HEU)**
高温化学处理【gāowēn huàxué chǔlǐ】	**pyrochemical processing**
高温气冷堆【gāowēn qìlěngduī】	**high temperature gas-cooled reactor (HTGR)**
高温冶金处理【gāowēn yějīn chǔlǐ】	**pyrometallurgical processing**
公报【gōngbào】	**communique**
公告【gōnggào】	**announcement**
公约【gōngyuē】	**convention**
供料【gōngliào】	**feed material**
供热反应堆【gōngrè fǎnyìngduī】	**nuclear heating reactor**
共同安全【gòngtóng ānquán】 冷战时期欧洲形成的一种安全概	**common security** A security concept that originated in Europe during the Cold War era. In

念。1982年，瑞典首相帕尔梅主持的“裁军和安全问题独立委员会”的报告《共同安全：生存蓝图》中首次提出。该报告认为，共同安全是基于这样一种认识，即安全的最佳保证是通过双边或多边的增强安全合作而非通过相互竞争的强权政治来获得。(源自：参考文献[1]，p23)	1982, the Independent Commission on Disarmament and Security Issues chaired by Swedish prime minister Olof Palme published a report entitled "Common Security: A Blueprint for Existence", which for the first time put forward this concept. The report pointed out that common security is based on the following concept: the best guarantee for security is obtained through cooperation in improving security for both or all parties rather than through competitive power politics.(From: Reference [1], p23)
钴弹【gǔdàn】 参见“感生放射性弹”	**cobalt bomb** Refer to "**induced-radioactivity bomb**"
关键测量点【guānjiàn cèliángdiǎn】	**key measurement point (KMP)**
关于朝鲜半岛无核化共同宣言 【guānyú cháoxiǎn bàndǎo wúhéhuà gòngtóng xuānyán】	**(North-South) Joint Declaration on the Denuclearization of the Korean Peninsula**
关于国际关系中不得进行武力威胁或使用武力的原则宣言 【guānyú guójìguānxì zhōng bùdé jìnxíng wǔlì wēixié huò shǐyòng wǔlì de yuánzé xuānyán】	**Principled Declaration on Refraining from the Threat or Use of Force in Their International Relations**
关于核材料、规定设备和非核材料自愿报告机制 【guānyú hécáiliào guīdìngshèbèi hé fēihécáiliào zìyuàn bàogào jīzhì】	**voluntary reporting scheme on nuclear material and specified equipment and non-nuclear material**
惯性约束聚变 【guànxìng yuēshù jùbiàn】	**inertial confinement fusion (ICF)**
罐装组件【guànzhuāng zǔjiàn】 核武器的次级装置，其内包含聚变燃料和(大多数情况下)铀装料(可能部分或全部是高浓铀)。(源自：参考文献[11]，p90)	**canned subassembly (CSA)** The secondary assembly in a nuclear weapon containing both fusion fuel and in most cases uranium (some or all of which may be HEU). (From: Reference [11], p90)

注：在美国，要装入最终武器的部件被称为“罐装组件”。	Note: In America, the subassembly that is to be incorporated into the final weapon is called a “canned subassembly”.
规定的设备【guīdìng de shèbèi】	**specified equipment**
规约【guīyuē】	**statute**
国防白皮书【guófáng báipíshū】	**Defense White Paper**
国际冲突【guójì chōngtū】	**international conflict**
国际法【guójìfǎ】	**international law**
国际惯例【guójì guànlì】	**international custom**
国际海事组织【guójì hǎishì zǔzhī】	**International Maritime Organization (IMO)**
国际衡算标准【guójì héngsuàn biāozhǔn】	**international standards of accountancy**
国际技术手段(核查用)【guójì jìshù shǒuduàn hécháyòng】	**international technical means (for verification)**
国际监测系统【guójì jiāncè xìtǒng】为核查《全面禁止核试验条约》(CTBT)执行情况而建立的核查机制的一个组成部分。它主要由地震监测网、大气放射性核素监测网、次声监测网和水声监测网组成。(源自：参考文献[1]，p478)	**International Monitoring System (IMS)** Part of the verification system that was established to verify the implementation of the Comprehensive Nuclear Test Ban Treaty (CTBT). It mainly consists of a seismic monitoring network, an atmospheric radionuclide monitoring network, an infrasound monitoring network and a hydroacoustic monitoring network. (From: Reference [1], p478)
国际经济新秩序【guójì jīngjì xīnzhìxù】	**new international economic order**
国际数据中心【guójì shùjù zhōngxīn】	**International Data Center (IDC)**
国际条约【guójì tiáoyuē】	**international treaty**
国际原子能机构【guójì yuánzǐnéng jīgòu】	**International Atomic Energy Agency (IAEA)**

国际原子能机构“93+2”计划 【guójì yuánzǐnéng jīgòu “93+2” jìhuà】	**IAEA's 93+2 program**
国际原子能机构保障监督的范围 【guójì yuánzǐnéng jīgòu bǎozhàng jiāndū de fànwéi】	**coverage of IAEA safeguards**
国际原子能机构保障监督的豁免 【guójì yuánzǐnéng jīgòu bǎozhàng jiāndū de huòmiǎn】	**exemption from IAEA safeguards**
国际原子能机构保障监督的起点 【guójì yuánzǐnéng jīgòu bǎozhàng jiāndū de qǐdiǎn】	**starting point of IAEA safeguards**
国际原子能机构保障监督的中止 【guójì yuánzǐnéng jīgòu bǎozhàng jiāndū de zhōngzhǐ】	**suspension of IAEA safeguards**
国际原子能机构保障监督的终止 【guójì yuánzǐnéng jīgòu bǎozhàng jiāndū de zhōngzhǐ】	**termination of IAEA safeguards**
国际原子能机构保障监督制度 【guójì yuánzǐnéng jīgòu bǎozhàng jiāndū zhìdù】 IAEA 的保障监督制度是 IAEA 为核实某国家履行未将民用核计划转用于核武器目的的国际承诺的一整套行动。保障监督体系是基于某国就其核材料和相关核活动向 IAEA 申报的准确性和完整性的评估。迄今为止，已有 145 个国家加入 IAEA 的保障监督协议，将核材料、核设施和核活动呈交 IAEA 保障监督视查员进行详细审查。IAEA 的核查有助于确认上述项目未转用或滥用于制造核武器，以及保障监督所要求申报的项目已全部申报。(源自：	**Safeguards of International Atomic Energy Agency** IAEA safeguards are a set of activities by which the IAEA seeks to verify that a State is living up to its international undertakings not to use peaceful nuclear programs for nuclear weapons purposes. The safeguards system is based on assessment of the correctness and completeness of the State's declarations to the IAEA concerning nuclear material and nuclear-related activities. To date, 145 States have entered into such agreements with the IAEA, submitting nuclear materials, facilities and activities to the scrutiny of IAEA's safeguards inspectors. IAEA verification helps to provide assurance that such items are not diverted or misused in

汉—英

汉—英

参考文献[51])	order to assemble nuclear weapons and that no items required to be declared under safeguards are undeclared. (From: Reference[51])
国际原子能机构的保障监督体系【guójì yuánzǐnéng jīgòu de bǎozhàng jiāndū tǐxì】	**IAEA Safeguards System**
国际原子能机构规约【guójì yuánzǐnéng jīgòu guīyuē】	**Statute of the International Atomic Energy Agency**
国际原子能机构及时性探知指标【guójì yuánzǐnéng jīgòu jíshíxìng tànzhī zhǐbiāo】	**IAEA timeliness detection goal**
国际原子能机构视察指标【guójì yuánzǐnéng jīgòu shìchá zhǐbiāo】	**IAEA inspection goal**
国际原子能机构特权和豁免协定【guójì yuánzǐnéng jīgòu tèquán hé huòmiǎn xiédìng】	**Agreement on the Privileges and Immunities of the IAEA**
国际战略格局【guójì zhànlüè géjú】	**international strategic pattern**
国际争端【guójì zhēngduān】	**international dispute**
国际政治新秩序【guójì zhèngzhì xīnzhìxù】	**new international political order**
国际制裁【guójì zhìcái】	**international sanction**
国家安全战略【guójiā ānquán zhànlüè】发展、运用和协调各种国家力量手段以实现有助于维护国家安全的目标。在美国，这是一个正式的官方文件。(改自：参考文献[9]，p367)	**national security strategy** Development, application, and coordination of the instruments of national power to achieve objectives that contribute to national security. In the U.S., it is a formal U.S. government document. (Modified from: Reference [9], p 367)
国家点火装置【guójiā diǎnhuǒ zhuāngzhì】	**National Ignition Facility (NIF)**
国家核材料衡算和控制系统【guójiā hécáiliào héngsuàn hé kòngzhì xìtǒng】	**state system of accounting for and control of nuclear material (SSAC)**

国家级保障监督方案 【guójiājí bǎozhàng jiāndū fāng'àn】 为具体国家制定的保障监督方案，方案涵盖该国所有与核材料、核设施以及与核燃料循环相关的活动。(源自：参考文献[4]，3.4)	**state-level safeguards approach** A safeguards approach developed for a specific State, encompassing all nuclear material, nuclear installations and nuclear fuel cycle related activities in that State. (From: Reference [4], 3.4)
国家技术手段 【guójiā jìshù shǒuduàn】 1 一个国家单方面拥有的核查和监测技术或措施，所获信息独家享用，常用于获取其他国家的相关活动的信息或情报。有时，也可用于军备控制条约或协议，以了解和核查其他参约方的遵约情况。(改自：参考文献[1]，p472) 2 在未侵入协议方领土、领空、领海的前提下，国家拥有的用于核查其他协议方是否遵约的手段。来自 NTM 的信息可用于国际核查制度，由条约缔约国向另一方质疑是否遵约。(源自：参考文献[19]，p198)	**national technical means (NTMs)** 1 Verification and monitoring technologies or measures owned by a country alone, and information thus collected will be used by itself. NTM is usually used to obtain information or intelligence on relevant activities conducted by other countries. It may also be used for understanding and verifying compliance with treaties or agreements related to arms control by other treaty signatories. (Modified from: Reference [1], p472) 2 NTM refers to nationally owned instruments for surveying a party's compliance with agreement obligations, without intruding onto its territory, airspace or national waters. Information derived from NTM may be used in international verification regimes by a treaty party to question another party's compliance. (From: Reference [19], p198)
国家军事战略【guójiā jūnshì zhànlüè】 分配和运用军事力量以实现国家安全战略和国防战略目标。(改自：参考文献[9]，p365)	**national military strategy** The deployment and application of military power to attain national security strategy and national defense strategy objectives. (Modified from: Reference [9], p365)
国家利益【guójiā lìyì】	**national interest**

国家战略【guójiā zhànlüè】	**national strategy**
海军用反应堆 【hǎijūnyòng fǎnyìngduī】	**naval reactor**
海洋监视卫星 【hǎiyáng jiānshì wèixīng】	**ocean surveillance satellite**
氦-3【hài sān】	**helium-3**
合成孔径雷达 【héchéng kǒngjìng léidá】	**synthetic aperture radar (SAR)**
合计铀【héjì yóu】	**unified uranium**
“合理足够”原则 【hélǐ zúgòu yuánzé】	**doctrine of "reasonable sufficiency"**
合作安全【hézuò ānquán】 冷战后形成的一种新的安全途径，“它强调安全保证，而不是威慑；它是包容性的，而不是排斥性的；它注重多边主义而不是单边或双边主义；它不认为军事手段高于非军事手段；它认为国家是安全体系里的主要行为体，但也接受非国家行为体能发挥重要作用；它不特别强调，但也不拒绝建立正式的安全机构；最重要的是，它强调建立对话习惯的重要性。”(源自：参考文献[65])	**cooperative security** A new security approach that evolved after the end of the Cold War, “which emphasizes reassurance rather than deterrence; it is inclusive rather than exclusive; favours multilateralism over unilateralism or bilateralism; does not rank military solutions over non-military ones; assumes that states are the principal actors in the security system but accepts that non-state actors have an important role to play; does not particularly emphasize the creation of formal security institutions, but does not reject them either; and which, above all, stresses the value of creating habits of dialogue.” (From: Reference [65])
合作减少威胁计划/纳恩-卢格计划 【hézuò jiǎnshǎo wēixié jìhuà nà'ēn lúgé jìhuà】 由美国国会于 1991 年 11 月通过。该立法授权国防部为符合条件的前苏联国家拆除和销毁大规模杀伤性武器提供资金援助，加强拆卸过程	**Cooperative Threat Reduction Program/Nunn-Lugar Program** The November 1991 legislation that provides the Department of Defense (DOD) with the authority to fund assistance to the eligible states of the former Soviet Union to dismantle and

中核武器和裂变材料的安全，防止扩散，帮助独联体国家(NIS)把大规模杀伤性武器的工业和科技基础设施转化为非军事目的。从 1996 年起，美国国务院负责武器专家的转行和出口控制，能源部负责核材料的控制和衡算。(改自：参考文献[50])	destroy weapons of mass destruction; to strengthen the security of nuclear weapons and fissile materials in connection with dismantlement; to prevent proliferation; and to help demilitarize the industrial and scientific infrastructure in the Newly Independent States (NIS) which has supported weapons of mass destruction. Since 1996, the Department of State and Department of Energy have assumed responsibility respectively for redirection of weapons expertise and export controls (State) and nuclear material control and accountability (DOE) program activities. (Modified from: Reference [50])
合作议定书【hézuò yìdìngshū】	**cooperation protocol**
和平共处五项原则 **【hépíng gòngchǔ wǔxiàng yuánzé】** 和平共处五项原则，即相互尊重主权和领土完整、互不侵犯、互不干涉内政、平等互利、和平共处。这五项原则由周恩来总理在与印度代表团谈判时提出，并于 1954 年 6 月首次被写入周恩来总理与贾瓦哈·尼赫鲁总理签署的联合公报中，此后被众多国际性文件所采用并成为公认的指导国际关系的准则。(源自：参考文献[53])	**Five Principles of Peaceful Coexistence** The Five Principles are: mutual respect for sovereignty and territorial integrity, mutual non-aggression, non-interference in each other's internal affairs, equality and mutual benefit, and peaceful coexistence. In negotiation with an Indian delegation the Five Principles were set forth by Premier Zhou Enlai, and subsequently included in the joint communique issued by Premier Zhou Enlai and Prime Minister Jawaharlal Nehru, in June 1954. Since that time the principles have been adopted in many other international documents. (Modified from: Reference[53])
和平核爆炸【hépíng hébàozhà】	**peaceful nuclear explosions**

和平解决理论【hépíng jiějué lǐlùn】	**theory of peaceful settlement**
和平利用核爆炸 【hépíng lìyòng hébàozhà】	**peaceful use of nuclear explosion**
核(爆炸)装置全过程数值模拟实验 【hé bàozhà zhuāngzhì quánguòchéng shùzhí mónǐ shíyàn】	**integrated numerical simulation experiment of explosion device**
核安全公约【hé'ānquán gōngyuē】	**Nuclear Safety Convention**
核爆材料【hébào cáiliào】 以适当的数量、纯度和构型存在时，能用以支持链式反应的核炸药和其他核素的混合物。(源自：参考文献[11]，p221)	**nuclear-explosive material (NEM)** Any mixture of nuclear-explosive and other nuclides that can be made to support a chain reaction when present in suitable quantity, purity, and geometry is called “nuclear-explosive material” (NEM). (From: Reference [11], p221)
核爆激励 X 射线激光器 【hébào jīlì X shèxiàn jīguāngqì】	**X-ray laser pumped by nuclear explosion**
核爆激励定向能武器 【hébào jīlì dìngxiàngnéng wǔqì】	**directed-energy weapon driven by a nuclear explosion**
核爆激励高功率微波武器 【hébào jīlì gāogōnglǜ wēibō wǔqì】 一种具有特殊性能的核爆炸装置，它通过与微波发生器耦合的方式，产生以高功率微波干扰或毁坏敌方通信系统或武器的电子部件。又称核爆驱动电磁脉冲弹。它是提议中第三代核武器的一种。(改自：参考文献[2]，p176)	**nuclear-explosion-driven microwave weapon** A nuclear explosive with special characteristics coupled with a special microwave generator that can disturb or destroy enemies' communication system or electronic components of weapons by high-power microwaves. It is one of the proposed third generation nuclear weapons. (Modified from: Reference [2], p176)
核爆驱动电磁脉冲弹 【hébào qūdòng diàncí màichōngdàn】	**electromagnetic pulse weapon driven by nuclear explosion**
核爆炸【hébàozhà】 利用能自持进行的原子核裂变或/和聚变反应瞬时释放的巨大能量，	**nuclear explosion** The process of producing explosive effects and potentially huge casualties

产生爆炸作用和可能造成巨大杀伤破坏效应的过程。(改自：参考文献[3]，p394) 注：核爆炸指由于在材料中发生自持裂变链式反应或裂变－聚变反应而导致材料解体(从纯粹的核聚变中获得能量的惯性约束聚变系统除外)。核反应堆，即使是裂变过程由于固体材料热膨胀而终止的脉冲核反应堆，也不属于核爆炸。(改自：参考文献[59]，p14-15)	and damage by huge energy instantaneously released from selfsustaining nuclear fission or/and fusion. (Modified from: Reference [3], p394) Note: A nuclear explosion is a self-sustaining fission chain reaction (or fission-fusion reaction) in a material that is disrupted in the process, with the exception of inertial-confinement fusion systems for obtaining energy from pure nuclear fusion. A nuclear reactor, even a pulsed nuclear reactor in which the fission process is terminated by thermal expansion of solid material, is not a nuclear explosion. (Modified from: Reference [59], p14-15)
核爆炸产生的放射性核素 【hébàozhà chǎnshēng de fàngshèxìng hésù】	**radioactive nuclide from nuclear explosion**
核爆炸产生的放射性气溶胶 【hébàozhà chǎnshēng de fàngshèxìng qìróngjiāo】	**radioactive aerosol of nuclear explosion**
核爆炸成坑效应 【hébàozhà chéngkēng xiàoyìng】	**cratering of nuclear explosion**
核爆炸冲击波【hébàozhà chōngjībō】	**nuclear explosion shock wave**
核爆炸的长期生物效应 【hébàozhà de chángqī shēngwù xiàoyìng】	**long-term biological effects of nuclear explosion**
核爆炸的计算机模拟 【hébàozhà de jìsuànjī mónǐ】	**computer simulation of a nuclear explosion**
核爆炸地球物理效应 【hébàozhà dìqiúwùlǐ xiàoyìng】	**geophysical effects of nuclear explosion**
核爆炸方式(环境) 【hébàozhà fāngshì huánjìng】 核武器或核爆炸装置在不同介质、	**type (environment) of nuclear explosion** Nuclear weapons or nuclear explosive

汉—英

不同高度或深度的爆炸，包括大气层核爆炸、高空核爆炸、水下核爆炸和地下核爆炸等。(改自：参考文献[1]，p191)	devices can be exploded in different media or at different heights/depths, in the atmosphere, in space, underwater and underground. (Modified from: Reference [1], p191)
核爆炸光(热)辐射【hébàozhà guāngrèfúshè】	**thermal radiation of nuclear explosion**
核爆炸光(热)辐射毁伤效应【hébàozhà guāngrèfúshè huǐshāng xiàoyìng】	**damaging and injuring effects of thermal radiation of nuclear explosion**
核爆炸环境取样【hébàozhà huánjìng qǔyàng】	**environmental sampling of nuclear explosion**
核爆炸火球【hébàozhà huǒqiú】	**nuclear explosion fireball**
核爆炸火球参数测量【hébàozhà huǒqiú cānshù cèliáng】	**measurement of nuclear fireball parameters**
核爆炸级瞬时辐射模拟源【hébàozhàjí shùnshí fúshè mónǐ yuán】	**nuclear-explosion-level prompt radiation simulation source**
核爆炸模拟【hébàozhà mónǐ】	**simulation of nuclear explosion**
核爆炸碎片的分凝【hébàozhà suìpiàn de fēnníng】	**nuclear explosion debris fractionation**
核爆炸探测【hébàozhà tàncè】	**detection of nuclear explosion**
核爆炸探测技术【hébàozhà tàncè jìshù】	**detection technology of nuclear explosion**
核爆炸探测系统【hébàozhà tàncè xìtǒng】	**detection system of nuclear explosion**
核爆炸通信效应【hébàozhà tōngxìn xiàoyìng】	**effects of nuclear explosion on communication**
核爆炸物理模拟【hébàozhà wùlǐ mónǐ】	**physical-simulation of nuclear explosion**
核爆炸现场视察技术【hébàozhà xiànchǎng shìchá jìshù】	**technologies for on-site inspection of nuclear explosion**
核爆炸效应【hébàozhà xiàoyìng】	**nuclear explosion effects**

核爆炸效应参数测量 【hébàozhà xiàoyìng cānshù cèliáng】	**measurement of nuclear explosion effect parameters**
核爆炸效应模拟 【hébàozhà xiàoyìng mónǐ】 利用各种模拟手段研究核爆炸破坏机理以及对核爆炸效应的保护措施。(改自：参考文献[3]，p377)	**simulation of nuclear explosion effects** Using various simulating measures to research the destructive mechanisms and protective measures against the effects of a nuclear explosion. (Modified from: Reference [3], p377)
核爆炸早期核辐射 【hébàozhà zǎoqī héfúshè】	**initial nuclear radiation of nuclear explosion**
核爆炸早期核辐射毁伤效应 【hébàozhà zǎoqī héfúshè huǐshāng xiàoyìng】	**injuring and damaging effects of initial nuclear radiation of nuclear explosion**
核爆炸装置【hébàozhà zhuāngzhì】 具有核爆炸功能的裂变装置或热核装置。(改自：参考文献[3]，p379)	**nuclear explosive device** A fission or thermonuclear device capable of producing a nuclear explosion. (Modified from: Reference [3], p379)
核材料【hécáiliào】	**nuclear material**
核材料擦拭样品 【hécáiliào cāshì yàngpǐn】	**swipe samples of nuclear material**
核材料初期存量 【hécáiliào chūqī cúnliàng】 某一衡算周期开始时所拥有的材料量。初始实物存量应等于前次材料衡算周期中核材料的末期存量。(源自：参考文献[2]，p186)	**beginning inventory of nuclear material** The amount of nuclear material at the beginning of a balancing period. It should be equal to the inventory at the end of the last material balancing period. (From: Reference [2], p186)
核材料初始存量 【hécáiliào chūshǐ cúnliàng】	**initial physical inventory of nuclear material**
核材料封隔【hécáiliào fēnggé】	**containment of nuclear material**
核材料衡算活动 【hécáiliào héngsuàn huódòng】 设施运行者和国家核材料衡算和控制系统所采取的衡算核材料的行动，尤其是为满足 IAEA 和该国(或	**nuclear material accountancy** The practice of nuclear material accounting as implemented by the facility operator and the State system of accounting for and control of nuclear material (SSAC), inter alia, to satisfy the

国家集团)之间的保障监督协议的要求，也包括 IAEA 所采取的类似行动，尤其是为独立核查国家核材料衡算和控制系统(SSAC)向 IAEA 所提供的设施纪录和报告中核材料衡算信息的正确性。(源自：参考文献[4]，6.2)	requirements in the safeguards agreement between the IAEA and the State (or group of States); and as implemented by the IAEA, inter alia, to independently verify the correctness of the nuclear material accounting information in the facility records and the reports provided by the SSAC to the IAEA. (From: Reference [4], 6.2)
核材料监视【hécáiliào jiānshì】	**surveillance of nuclear material**
核材料末期存量 **【hécáiliào mòqī cúnliàng】**	**ending inventory of nuclear material**
核材料平衡区【hécáiliào pínghéngqū】	**material balance area (MBA)**
核材料实体保护 **【hécáiliào shítǐ bǎohù】** 对存有核材料的建筑物和车辆(涉及储存和运输过程)等建立安全防范系统，以实施对核材料的保障监督。(源自：参考文献[2]，p186)	**physical-protection for nuclear material** Establishing a security protection system for extant buildings and vehicles (relating to storage or transportation processes) with nuclear material, so as to safeguard nuclear material. (From: Reference [2], p186)
核材料实体保护等级 **【hécáiliào shítǐ bǎohù děngjí】**	**physical-protection levels of nuclear material**
核材料实体保护授权 **【hécáiliào shítǐ bǎohù shòuquán】**	**physical-protection authorization of nuclear material**
核材料实体(物)保护公约 **【hécáiliào shítǐwù bǎohù gōngyuē】** 该公约以促进《不扩散核武器条约》的各缔约国和平发展和利用核能为目的，并加强各国对核材料使用、储存和运输的保护，防止核材料的非法获取及使用而可能造成的危险。公约于 1980 年 3 月签署。2005 年 7 月通过了旨在进一步加强核设	**Convention on Physical Protection for Nuclear Material** The convention signed to promote the peaceful purpose of developing and using nuclear energy among every Nuclear Nonproliferation Treaty State Party, to strengthen the protection of nuclear material usage, storage and transportation, and to prevent the possible dangers caused by illegally obtaining and using nuclear material. It was signed on 3 March, 1980. In July

施与核材料保护的公约修订案并签署了新公约。新公约采纳了中国提交的支持国际社会加强对核设施保护的努力、反对以任何形式对其他国家和平核设施动用武力或进行武力威胁的修订案。新公约还首次明确规定，缔约国要在保护核材料安全、防范核恐怖主义方面进一步加强国际合作。(源自：参考文献[52])	2005, the amended version of the convention that aims to further strengthen the protection of nuclear material and facilities was adopted and the new convention was signed. The new convention accepted the amendment submitted by China which declared its support for the effort of the International community to strengthen the protection of nuclear facilities, and opposed any form of force or threat of force to any States' peaceful nuclear facility. It also prescribes for the first time that any State Party should further strengthen international cooperation on protecting the safety of nuclear material and preventing nuclear terrorism. (From: Reference[52])
核材料实物盘存 【hécáiliào shíwù páncún】 为确定核材料实物存量而采取的行动。(改自：参考文献[15]，para113；[4]，6.41)	**physical inventory-taking of nuclear material** The activities carried out to determine physical inventory. (Modified from: Reference [15], para113; [4], 6.41)
核材料现有库存 【hécáiliào xiànyǒu kùcún】	**existing stock of nuclear material**
核材料意外事件 【hécáiliào yìwài shìjiàn】	**nuclear material incident**
核材料转化时间 【hécáiliào zhuǎnhuà shíjiān】	**conversion time of nuclear material**
核材料转用 【hécáiliào zhuǎnyòng】	**diversion of nuclear material**
核查【héchá】 在军控中是指确认缔约国是否遵守协议条款的过程。它必须监测各缔约国有关条约承诺的活动，分析从	**verification** In the arms control field, it refers to the process of establishing whether state parties are complying with the provision of an agreement. It entails monitoring

汉-英

监测收集的信息，并确定各缔约国是否遵守其对条约承诺的义务。(改自：参考文献[19]，p237)	the activities of the parties relevant to their treaty commitments, analysing the information collected from monitoring, and determining whether the parties are complying with their agreement obligations. (Modified from: Reference [19], p237)
核出口控制【héchūkǒu kòngzhì】 对核材料、核设备和反应堆用非核材料等物项及其相关技术的贸易性出口及对外赠送、展览、科技合作和援助进行控制。(改自：参考文献[25])	**nuclear export control** Control of commercial export, gifts to and exhibitions in foreign countries or regions, as well as scientific and technological cooperation with and assistance to foreign countries or regions that involve nuclear materials, nuclear equipment, non-nuclear materials used for reactors and other items as well as their related technologies. (Modified from: Reference [25])
核打击【hédǎjī】	**nuclear strike**
核打击目标【hédǎjī mùbiāo】	**target of nuclear strike**
核弹头再入遥测【hédàntóu zàirù yáocè】	**reentry telemetry for nuclear reentry vehicle**
核导弹弹头【hédǎodàn dàntóu】 1 装有核战斗部的导弹再入飞行器。(源自：参考文献[3]，p96) 2 再入飞行器——设计为再入地球大气层的空间飞行器部件。(源自：参考文献[9]，p456) 3 再入飞行器(或(再入)弹头)——在导弹的弹道终端能再入地球大气层的弹道导弹上的核战斗部。(源自：参考文献[8]) 注：“再入飞行器”的一种非常用	**nuclear missile reentry vehicle** 1 A missile reentry vehicle equipped with a nuclear warhead. (From: Reference [3], p96) 2 reentry vehicle (RV)——The part of a space vehicle designed to re-enter the earth's atmosphere. (From: Reference [9], p456) 3 reentry vehicle (RV)——A nuclear warhead on a ballistic missile specially designed to reenter the earth's atmosphere in the terminal portion of the missile's trajectory. (From: Reference [8]) Note: The term “reentry body” is the

名称是“再入体”。	less-common equivalent of “reentry vehicle”.
核导弹的戒备率 【hédǎodàn de jièbèilǜ】 处于各种戒备状态并能在规定发射准备时间内实施作战发射的导弹数占部署导弹总数的百分比。(改自：参考文献[2]，p49)	**alert rate of nuclear missiles** The percentage of those missiles that are on various stages of alert and can launch in stipulated preparatory times in relation to the entire arsenal of deployed missiles. (Modified from: Reference [2], p49)
核导弹的突防装置 【hédǎodàn de tūfáng zhuāngzhì】	**penetration aids of nuclear missiles**
核导弹反应时间 【hédǎodàn fǎnyìng shíjiān】 核导弹从接到发射命令到导弹起飞所需的时间。(源自：参考文献[2]，p50)	**response time of nuclear missiles** The time elapsed from receiving launch orders to the launch of nuclear missiles. (From: Reference [2], p50)
核导弹可靠性【hédǎodàn kěkàoxìng】	**reliability of nuclear missiles**
核导弹射程【hédǎodàn shèchéng】	**range of nuclear missiles**
核导弹投掷重量 【hédǎodàn tóuzhì zhòngliàng】	**throw weight of nuclear missile**
核电厂废物【hédiànchǎng fèiwù】	**waste from nuclear power plant**
核电磁脉冲【hédiàncí màichōng】	**nuclear electromagnetic pulse (NEMP)**
核电磁脉冲的传播 【hédiàncímàichōng de chuánbō】	**propagation of nuclear electromagnetic pulse**
核电磁脉冲的防护 【hédiàncí màichōng de fánghù】	**protection from nuclear electromagnetic pulse**
核冬天【hédōngtiān】	**nuclear winter**
核讹诈【hé’ézhà】	**nuclear blackmail**
核反击【héfǎnjī】	**nuclear counterattack**
核反应【héfǎnyìng】	**nuclear reaction**
核供应国集团【hégōngyìngguó jítuán】 通过执行核(和涉及核)出口准则而	**Nuclear Suppliers Group (NSG)** A group of nuclear supplier countries which seeks to contribute to the

汉-英

防止核武器扩散的核供应国家。各参与国通过其国家法律和惯例来执行核供应国集团的准则。出口申请由国家层面决定，并符合国家出口许可规定。(源自：参考文献[47])	non-proliferation of nuclear weapons through the implementation of Guide-lines for nuclear exports and nuclear related exports. The NSG Guidelines are implemented by each Participating Government in accordance with its national laws and practices. Decisions on export applications are taken at the national level in accordance with national export licensing requirements. (From: Reference [47])
核供应国集团准则【hégōngyìngguó jítuán zhǔnzé】	**Nuclear Suppliers Group Guidelines**
核黑匣子【hé hēixiázi】 装有总统用来授权使用战略核武器的指令和密码的便携手提箱或手提包的俗称。(改自：参考文献[2]，p203)	**nuclear football** A popular name of a portable briefcase or package that contains instructions and codes for the president to authorize the use of strategic nuclear weapons. (Modified from: Reference[2], p203)
核裂变【hélièbiàn】	**nuclear fission**
核门槛国家【héménkǎn guójiā】	**nuclear threshold state (NTS)**
核能级【hénéngjí】	**nuclear energy level**
核炮弹【hépàodàn】	**nuclear artillery projectile**
核燃料【héránliào】	**nuclear fuel**
核燃料后处理【héránliào hòuchǔlǐ】	**nuclear fuel reprocessing**
核燃料循环【héránliào xúnhuán】 由与核材料物流相关的核设施及核活动组成的系统。从由国外提供带燃料的单个反应堆，到一整套完善系统，不同国家之间燃料循环的特点可能存在很大差异。(源自：参考文献[4]，4.30)	**nuclear fuel cycle** A system of nuclear installations and activities interconnected by streams of nuclear material. The characteristics of the fuel cycle may vary widely from State to State, from a single reactor supplied from abroad with fuel, to a fully developed system. (From: Reference[4], 4.30)
核燃料循环废物【héránliào xúnhuán fèiwù】	**waste from nuclear fuel cycle**

汉—英

核深水炸弹【hé shēnshuǐ zhàdàn】	**nuclear depth bomb**
核试验【héshìyàn】	**nuclear test**
核试验测试技术 【héshìyàn cèshì jìshù】	**measurement technology of nuclear test**
核试验场【héshìyànchǎng】	**nuclear test site**
核试验的物理诊断测量 【héshìyàn de wùlǐzhěnduàn cèliáng】	**physical diagnostic measurement in nuclear test**
核试验的诊断和测量 【héshìyàn de zhěnduàn hé cèliáng】	**diagnostic and measurement of nuclear test**
核试验放射化学诊断 【héshìyàn fàngshèhuàxué zhěnduàn】	**radiochemical diagnostic of nuclear test**
核衰变【héshuāibiàn】	**nuclear decay**
核素【hésù】	**nuclide**
核损耗【hésǔnhào】 指由于核反应使核材料转变成其他元素或同位素而造成的核材料损耗。核损耗还包括核材料在反应堆中燃烧所造成的损耗以及存储期间衰变所造成的损耗(例如钚-241 的衰变)。(源自：参考文献[4]，6.22)	**nuclear loss** Loss of nuclear material due to its transformation into other element(s) or isotope(s) as a result of nuclear reactions. Nuclear loss also includes burn up of nuclear material in a reactor and decay (e.g. of Pu-241) during storage. (From: Reference [4], 6.22)
核威慑【héwēishè】 以给觉察到的或潜在的敌人造成无法承受的毁伤的核报复相威胁，从而防止敌人实施核打击的战略。(源自：参考文献[6]，p177) 注：原则上，核威慑不仅仅可以用来阻止核攻击，而且也可以用来阻止常规力量、化学或生物武器的攻击，甚至用来阻止由非军事手段使至关重要的国家利益遭受损害的攻击。 (源自：参考文献[7]，p14-15)	**nuclear deterrence** A strategy of preventing a nuclear attack by threatening the perceived or potential enemy with unacceptable damage by nuclear retaliation. (From: Reference [6], p177) Note: In principle, nuclear deterrence could be used to deter not only nuclear attacks but also attacks with conventional forces, attacks with chemical or biological weapons, or even assaults on vital national interests by nonmilitary means. (From: Reference [7], p14-15)

核威胁【héwēixié】	**nuclear threat**
核武库维护与管理计划 【héwǔkù wéihù yǔ guǎnlǐ jìhuà】	**Stockpile Stewardship and Management Program**
核武器【héwǔqì】 1 利用能自持进行的原子核裂变和(或)聚变反应瞬时释放的巨大能量，产生爆炸作用，并具有大规模毁伤破坏效应的武器。从广义上说它是指包括投掷或发射系统在内的具有作战能力的核武器系统。(改自：参考文献[3]，p394) 2 北约定义——根据预期设计构造，在完成指定的引爆控制序列后，能够产生预期的核反应并释放出核能的完整装置(如内爆型、枪型或热核型)。也被称为“原子武器”。(源自：参考文献[49]，p11) 3 俄罗斯定义——俄罗斯联邦军队的核武器是指包括核装料、核战斗部、运载工具和控制系统在内的武器系统。(源自：参考文献[29]，p21) 4 使原子核产生裂变或聚变链式反应(或兼而有之)，以爆炸方式释放核能的装置。(源自：参考文献[8])	**nuclear weapon** 1 Weapon assembly that is capable of producing an explosion and massive injury and destruction by the sudden release of energy instantaneously released from self-sustaining nuclear fission and/or fusion. From the generalized point of view, it refers to nuclear weapon system with a warfighting capability including the delivery or launch system. (Modified from: Reference [3], p394) 2 NATO definition — A complete assembly (i.e. implosion type, gun type or thermonuclear type) in its intended ultimate configuration which, upon completion of the prescribed arming, fusing and firing sequence, is capable of producing the intended nuclear reaction and release of energy. Also called “atomic weapon”. (From: Reference [49], p11) 3 Russian definition — Nuclear Weapons in the Armed Forces of the Russian Federation include an aggregate of armaments including nuclear charges, nuclear ammunition, means of their delivery to the target and control means. (From: Reference [29], p21) 4 A device that releases nuclear energy in an explosive manner as the result of nuclear chain reactions involving the fission or fusion, or both, of atomic nuclei. (From: Reference [8])

核武器安全性【héwǔqì ānquánxìng】 在正常的维护或使用核武器中，防止因设备或武器的误操作、逐步退化或意外故障等原因发生人员、设备和设施的事故的能力。(改自：参考文献[2]，p217)	**nuclear weapon safety** In maintenance and use of nuclear weapons, the capability to avoid an accident involving personnel, facilities and installations due to misuse or from gradual deterioration or a sudden fault in equipment or weapons. (Modified from: Reference [2], p217)
核武器保安性【héwǔqì bǎo'ānxìng】 核武器及其相关的设备和人员能抵制任何非授权的使用的能力。(改自：参考文献[2]，p217)	**nuclear weapon security** The capability of a nuclear weapon and its surrounding equipment and personnel to prevent any unauthorized use. (Modified from: Reference [2], p217)
核武器保险装置 【héwǔqì bǎoxiǎn zhuāngzhì】 参见“密码锁(亦称启动连接装置)”	**safing device of nuclear weapon** Refer to “**permissive action link (PAL)**”
核武器触发引信 【héwǔqì chùfā yǐnxìn】	**contact fuze of nuclear weapon**
核武器的防护 【héwǔqì de fánghù】	**protection of nuclear weapon**
核武器的延寿与退役 【héwǔqì de yánshòu yǔ tuìyì】	**lifetime extension and decommissioning of nuclear weapon**
核武器地面测控设备 【héwǔqì dìmiàn cèkòng shèbèi】	**equipment for ground test and monitoring of nuclear weapon**
核武器工程设计 【héwǔqì gōngchéng shèjì】	**engineering design of nuclear weapon**
核武器惯性引信 【héwǔqì guànxìng yǐnxìn】	**inertia fuze of nuclear weapon**
核武器国家【héwǔqì guójiā】	**nuclear weapon state (NWS)**
核武器环境模拟试验 【héwǔqì huánjìng mónǐ shìyàn】	**environmental simulation test of nuclear weapon**
核武器解保【héwǔqì jiěbǎo】	**arming nuclear weapon**
核武器可靠性【héwǔqì kěkàoxìng】 核武器在使用寿命期间，在规定的	**reliability of nuclear weapon** Throughout the nuclear weapon's

汉-英

正常环境条件下，以设计性能指标实现核爆炸的能力。(改自：参考文献，[2] p221) 注 1：在核武器的整个设计寿命期间，经受从库存至打击目标的各种外部环境，在正确输入指令后，能在打击目标上实现指定威力的概率。在此定义中，“指定威力”通常被理解成与设计威力相差 10%以内的意思；“从库存至打击目标的环境”指核弹头在其服役期内的储存、转运和使用过程中会经历的外部环境，如极端温度、核导弹防御拦截器的辐射、过载；“寿命”指在设计时指定的初始寿命目标；“正确输入”指引爆控制信号。(源自：参考文献[10]，p8) 注 2：圣地亚国家实验室的定义中，“武器”有“核弹头”的意思；如果“武器”有包含导弹或飞行器的“武器系统”的意思，那么可靠性将更低。	lifetime, the capability to achieve the nuclear explosion within the designed performance under the defined normal environment. (Modified from: Reference [2], p221) Note 1: The probability of achieving the specified yield, at the target, across the Stockpile-To-Target Sequence of environments, throughout the weapon's lifetime, assuming proper inputs. In this definition, the specified yield is generally understood to mean within ten percent; the Stockpile-To-Target Sequence of environments is the range of conditions the warhead is expected to experience in its service life in storage, transit, or use, such as temperature extremes, radiation from any nuclear-armed missile defense interceptors, and acceleration; lifetime is the "original lifetime objective as specified at the time of design"; and proper inputs are arming, fuzing, and firing signals. (From: Reference[10], p8.) Note 2: In this definition by Sandia National Laboratories, "weapon" has the meaning of "warhead"; if "weapon" had the meaning of "weapon system" including the missile or aircraft, the reliability would be much lower.
核武器可维修性 【héwǔqì kěwéixiūxìng】	**maintainability of nuclear weapon**
核武器库存【héwǔqì kùcún】	**nuclear weapons stockpile**
核武器雷达引信【héwǔqì léidá yǐnxìn】	**radar fuze of nuclear weapon**
核武器路程长度引信 【héwǔqì lùchéng chángdù yǐnxìn】	**path-length fuze of nuclear weapon**

核武器气压引信【héwǔqì qìyā yǐnxìn】	**atmospheric-pressure fuze of nuclear weapon**
核武器确信性 【héwǔqì quèxìnxìng】 使用能提高核武器安全性、保安性、可靠性和可控性的材料、人员和程序，以确保核武器在使用过程中不发生核事故、故障、非授权使用或功能退化。(源自：参考文献[60])	**nuclear weapons surety** The materiel, personnel, and procedures that contribute to the safety, security, reliability, and control of nuclear weapons, thus assuring no nuclear accidents, incidents, unauthorized use, or degradation in performance. (From: Reference [60])
核武器生存能力 【héwǔqì shēngcún nénglì】 一方的现役核武器在对方进行第一次核打击后保持完好的能力。(源自：参考文献[2]，p222)	**survivability of nuclear weapon** Capability for nuclear weapons on active service to remain intact after another country launches a first nuclear strike. (From: Reference [2], p222)
核武器事故【héwǔqì shìgù】	**nuclear weapon accidents**
核武器寿命【héwǔqì shòumìng】 核武器从出厂到无法满足技术性能指标和作战使用要求的整个过程的期限。(改自：参考文献[2]，p222)	**lifespan of nuclear weapon** The whole period of a nuclear weapon's life, beginning from when it was produced until when it could no longer fulfill technical performance criteria or meet operational requirements. (Modified from: Reference [2], p222)
核武器投射【héwǔqì tóushè】	**projection of nuclear weapon**
核武器突防能力 【héwǔqì tūfáng nénglì】	**penetration ability of nuclear weapon**
核武器物理【héwǔqì wùlǐ】	**nuclear weapon physics**
核武器小型化【héwǔqì xiǎoxínghuà】	**nuclear weapon miniaturization**
核武器遥测系统 【héwǔqì yáocè xìtǒng】	**telemetry system for nuclear weapon**
核武器一点安全 【héwǔqì yīdiǎn ānquán】 核武器在异常环境(撞击或枪击)下	**one-point safety of a nuclear weapon** Safety performance of a nuclear

武器中炸药任何一点起爆时所具有的安全性能。美国军用标准为：在任何事故中，炸药任何一点起爆时所产生的裂变能在 1.8 千克梯恩梯当量以上的概率小于百万分之一。(改自：参考文献[2]，p223)	weapon when any one point of the high explosive is detonated in abnormal situations (by impact, projectile, etc). The U.S. military standard is that the probability of releasing more than 1.8 kg TNT equivalent fission energy when any point of the explosive is ignited is less than one per million in any accident. (Modified from: Reference [2], p223)
核武器引爆【héwǔqì yǐnbào】	**firing the nuclear weapon**
核武器引信【héwǔqì yǐnxìn】	**fuze of nuclear weapon**
核武器用中子发生器【héwǔqìyòng zhōngzǐ fāshēngqì】	**neutron generator used in nuclear weapon**
核武器运用的运筹分析【héwǔqì yùnyòng de yùnchóu fēnxī】	**operations research and analysis of nuclear weapon employment**
核武器战术技术性能【héwǔqì zhànshù jìshù xìngnéng】	**operational characteristics of nuclear weapon**
核武器制胜论【héwǔqì zhìshènglùn】	**theory of victory decided by nuclear weapons**
核武器贮存环境【héwǔqì zhùcún huánjìng】	**storage environment of nuclear weapon**
核武器贮存期【héwǔqì zhùcúnqī】	**storage life of nuclear weapon**
核武器贮存与保管【héwǔqì zhùcún yǔ bǎoguǎn】	**storage and custody of nuclear weapon**
核武器装订爆高【héwǔqì zhuāngdìng bàogāo】	**preset burst height of nuclear weapon**
核武器装订爆深【héwǔqì zhuāngdìng bàoshēn】	**preset burst depth of nuclear weapon**
核武器自毁装置【héwǔqì zìhuǐ zhuāngzhì】	**self-destruct device of nuclear weapon**
核武器自相摧毁效应【héwǔqì zìxiāng cuīhuǐ xiàoyìng】	**fratricidal effect of nuclear weapon**
核武器总体设计【héwǔqì zǒngtǐ shèjì】	**overall design of nuclear weapon**

核武装力量【héwǔzhuāng lìliàng】	**nuclear forces**
核物质【héwùzhì】	**nuclear matter**
核相关两用物项 【hé xiāngguān liǎngyòng wùxiàng】 指一种在核和非核领域都有技术用途的物项，提供这种物项时要遵守一定条件，因为这种物项可能为核爆炸活动提供很大的帮助。(改自：参考文献[4]，5.34)	**nuclear-related dual-use item** An item which has a technical use in both nuclear and non-nuclear applications, and may be subject to certain conditions of supply because such items could make a major contribution to a nuclear explosive activity. (Modified from: Reference [4], 5.34)
核学说【héxuéshuō】 为支持国家战略目标而规定在何种情形下以何种方式使用核武器的基本原则。(改自：参考文献[9])	**nuclear doctrine** The fundamental principles governing the conditions under which and the modalities of how nuclear weapons are to be used in support of national objectives. (Modified from: Reference [9])
核优势【héyōushì】 一个核国家的核武器拥有明显的质量和数量上的优势足以阻止或摧毁对手的报复性(第二次)打击能力的状态。(改自：参考文献[22]) 注：另一种观点是，“摧毁对手所有核力量、消除报复性打击可能性的能力，被认为是一种第一次打击能力或核优势”。(源自：参考文献[22])	**nuclear primacy** The condition whereby one state holds a clear qualitative and quantitative ability to prevent or render ineffective a rival's retaliatory (second) strike capability. (Modified from: Reference [22]) Note: In another view, “The ability to destroy all of an adversary's nuclear forces, eliminating the possibility of a retaliatory strike, is known as a first-strike capability, or nuclear primacy.” (From: Reference [22])
核炸弹【hézhàdàn】	**nuclear bomb**
核战斗部【hézhàndòubù】 核武器中用来毁伤目标的部分。主要由核爆炸装置、引爆控制系统、其他功能部件和相应的结构部件等组成。在中国军备控制领域常把核	**nuclear warhead** The part of a nuclear weapon whose function is to destroy or damage targets. It mainly consists of a nuclear explosive device, arming, fuzing and firing system，and other functional parts or relevant structures. In Chinese

战斗部称为核弹头。(改自：参考文献[3]，p404) 注：战斗部——导弹、炮弹、鱼雷、火箭或其他武器的毁伤目标的部分，它含有核或热核系统、高能炸药系统、生物或化学制剂、或惰性材料。(源自：参考文献[5]，p15)	writings in the arms control field, the nuclear warhead is often called 【hédàntóu】(核弹头). (Modified from: Reference [3], p404) Note: The warhead is the part of a missile, projectile, torpedo, rocket, or other munition which contains either the nuclear or thermonuclear system, high explosive system, chemical or biological agents or inert materials intended to inflict damage. (From: Reference [5], p15)
核战略【hézhànlüè】 筹划和指导核力量发展与运用的方略。(源自：参考文献[1]，p112)	**nuclear strategy** Strategy of planning and guiding the development and employment of nuclear force. (From: Reference [1], p112)
核战能力【hézhàn nénglì】 在核战略中，具有使用核武器进行战争的能力，而不仅限于慑止核战争爆发的能力。(改自：参考文献[48])	**nuclear warfighting capability** In nuclear strategy, having the capability to use nuclear weapons to fight a war, and not just to deter the outbreak of nuclear war. (Modified from: Reference [48])
核战役【hézhànyì】 在一定时间和区域内为实现战役或战略目标所采取的一系列使用核武器的相关军事行动。(改自：参考文献[9]，p76)	**nuclear campaign** A series of related military operations using nuclear weapons aimed at accomplishing a strategic or operational objective within a given time and space. (Modified from: Reference [9], p76)
核战争【hézhànzhēng】	**nuclear war**
核子【hézǐ】	**nucleon**
核钻地弹【hézuāndìdàn】	**nuclear earth penetrator**
核作战计划【hézuòzhàn jìhuà】	**nuclear operation plan**
衡算记录【héngsuàn jìlù】	**accounting records**
红外遥感器【hóngwài yáogǎnqì】	**infrared remote sensor**
后处理【hòuchǔlǐ】	**reprocessing**

后处理厂【hòuchǔlǐ chǎng】	**reprocessing plant**
环境取样【huánjìng qǔyàng】 在 IAEA 保障监督框架内，从环境中取样，并通过对样品的分析获取相关痕迹以揭示所处理的核材料或进行的活动的信息。(源自：参考文献[4]，9.1)	**environmental sampling** In the context of IAEA safeguards, the collection of samples from the environment with a view to analyzing them for traces of materials that can reveal information about nuclear material handled or activities conducted. (From: Reference [4], 9.1)
缓和【huǎnhé】	**detente**
换文【huànwén】	**exchange of notes**
黄饼【huángbǐng】 铀水冶过程中的中间产物，含有大约 80%带着少量铀酰盐的八氧化三铀(U_3O_8)。用于铀浓缩的黄饼被转化成六氟化铀气体(UF_6)，用于天然铀反应堆燃料的黄饼被加工成纯净的二氧化铀。(源自：参考文献[12])	**yellow cake** A concentrate produced during the uranium milling process that contains about 80% U_3O_8 with small amounts of uranyl salts. In preparation for uranium enrichment, the yellowcake is converted to uranium hexafluoride gas (UF_6). In the preparation of natural uranium reactor fuel, yellowcake is processed into purified uranium dioxide. (From: Reference [12])
毁伤概率【huǐshāng gàilǜ】	**kill probability**
毁伤软目标能力【huǐshāng ruǎnmùbiāo nénglì】	**capability of destroying soft target**
毁伤硬目标能力【huǐshāng yìngmùbiāo nénglì】	**capability of destroying hardened target**
混合氧化物【hùnhé yǎnghuàwù】	**mixed oxide (MOX)**
混合样品【hùnhé yàngpǐn】	**composite sample**
机动导弹【jīdòng dǎodàn】	**mobile missile**
机动再入弹头【jīdòng zàirù dàntóu】	**maneuverable reentry vehicle (MaRV)**
积极防御【jījí fángyù】	**active defense** Note 1: Term used to describe China's

汉—英

注 1：用以描述中国军事战略的术语。它主要包括以下三方面的内容：一是坚持自卫立场和实行后发制人；二是以积极主动的军事准备和政治斗争防止战争；三是一旦战争爆发，以积极的反击和进攻作战达成战略防御目的。(改自：参考文献[31]，p124-125)	military strategy. It includes the following main elements: firstly, taking a firm stand of self-defense and gaining mastery by striking only after the enemy has struck; secondly, using active military preparations and political struggle to prevent war; thirdly, should war break out, using active counter-attack and offensive operations to achieve strategic defensive objectives. (Modified from: Reference [31], p124-125)
注 2：在美国，“积极防御”指采取有限的攻击及反击以防止敌方占领竞争中的区域或地点。(源自：参考文献[9]，p4) 注 3：在导弹防御领域，“积极防御”指拦截并摧毁导弹或其弹头；“消极防御”指主要通过使用爆炸掩体和食物存储等来抵御弹头的效用。(改自：参考文献[62])	Note 2: In the U.S., “active defense” is the employment of limited offensive action and counterattacks to deny a contested area or position to the enemy. (From: Reference [9], p4) Note 3: In the context of missile defense, “active defense” means the interception and destruction of missiles or their warheads; “passive defense” is protection against the effects of the warheads primarily by the use of blast shelters, stockpiling of food, etc. (Modified from: Reference [62])
基准数据视察【jīzhǔn shùjù shìchá】	**baseline data inspection**
激光等离子体离子萃取【jīguāng děnglízǐtǐlízǐ cuìqǔ】	**laser plasma ion extraction**
激光分离同位素【jīguāng fēnlí tóngwèisù】	**laser isotope separation**
激光化学法分离同位素【jīguāng huàxuéfǎ fēnlí tóngwèisù】	**laser chemical isotope separation**
级联【jílián】	**cascade**
级联理论【jílián lǐlùn】	**theory of cascade**
级联效率【jílián xiàolǜ】	**efficiency of cascade**
集体安全【jítǐ ānquán】	**collective security**

多国通过有组织的集体行动来预防和制止侵略，保护各国安全的一种方式。(源自：参考文献[1]，p23)	An approach to prevent and curb aggre-ssion and maintain security for countri-es through the organized collective action of multiple countries. (From: Reference [1], p23)
集体辐照剂量【jítǐ fúzhào jìliàng】	**collective radiation dose**
技术防护系统的多样性【jìshù fánghù xìtǒng de duōyàngxìng】	**diversity of technical protection systems**
技术防护系统的多重性【jìshù fánghù xìtǒng de duōchóngxìng】	**multiplicity of technical protection system**
技术特性展示和视察【jìshù tèxìng zhǎnshì hé shìchá】	**technical characteristics exhibition and inspection**
加固目标【jiāgù mùbiāo】	**hardened target**
加速战略计算倡议【jiāsù zhànlüè jìsuàn chàngyì】 注：现已改为“先进模拟与计算计划”。(源自：参考文献[37])	**Accelerated Strategic Computing Initiative (ASCI)** Note: The program has been changed to Advanced Simulation and Computing Program (ASC). (From: Reference [37])
价值函数【jiàzhí hánshù】	**value function**
监测【jiāncè】 为核查获取信息的途径。(源自：参考文献[16])	**monitoring** The means by which information is obtained for verification purposes. (From: Reference [16])
减威力核试验【jiǎnwēilì héshìyàn】	**reduced yield nuclear test**
建立信任与安全措施【jiànlì xìnrèn yǔ ānquán cuòshī】	**Confidence and Security Building Measures (CSBMs)**
舰船用动力反应堆【jiànchuányòng dònglì fǎnyìngduī】	**marine propulsion reactor**
校准【jiàozhǔn】	**calibration**
结合能【jiéhé’néng】	**binding energy**
解除豁免【jiěchú huòmiǎn 】	**de-exemption**
解耦的地下核爆炸【jiě’ǒu de dìxià hébàozhà】	**decoupled underground nuclear explosion**

金属钚【jīnshǔbù】	**metallic plutonium**
金属燃料【jīnshǔ ránliào】	**metallic fuel**
金属铀【jīnshǔyóu】	**metallic uranium**
近区物理诊断【jìnqū wùlǐ zhěnduàn】 直接测量核爆炸过程中伴随着核反应放出的中子、γ射线、X 射线，以判断核武器性能参数。(改自：参考文献[3]，p391)	**near-field physical diagnostic** To judge nuclear weapons' performance parameters by directly measuring neutrons, γ-rays, and X-rays released from the nuclear reactions. (Modified from: Reference [3], p391)
进攻性战略【jìngōngxìng zhànlüè】 为接近并摧毁敌方军事力量以及夺取疆土和重要资源而对敌方采取的军事行动。它致力于抢占、保持和发挥主动权。(源自：参考文献[61]，p3-27)	**offensive strategy** A strategy that aims to carry military operations to the enemy by closing with and destroying enemy forces, seizing territory and vital resources. Its focus is on seizing, retaining, and exploiting the initiative. (From: Reference [61], p3-27)
禁止【jìnzhǐ】	**ban**
禁止生产易裂变材料核查 【jìnzhǐ shēngchǎn yìlièbiàn cáiliào héchá】	**verification of the fissile material production cutoff**
禁止为核武器生产易裂变材料 【jìnzhǐ wèi héwǔqì shēngchǎn yìlièbiàn cáiliào】	**prohibition of the production of fissile material for nuclear weapon**
禁止在大气层、外层空间和水下进行核武器试验条约 【jìnzhǐ zài dàqìcéng wàicéng kōngjiān hé shuǐxià jìnxíng héwǔqì shìyàn tiáoyuē】	**Treaty Banning Nuclear Weapon Tests in the Atmosphere, in Outer Space and Under Water (PTBT)**
经典超级模型 【jīngdiǎn chāojí móxíng】	**classical super design**
旧核三位一体【jiù hé sānweìyītǐ】 美国战略核力量的三个支柱：潜射弹道导弹(SLBMs)；陆基洲际弹道导弹(ICBMs)；远程轰炸机。(源自：参考文献[72])	**old nuclear triad** The three legs of the U.S. strategic nuclear force: submarine-launched ballistic missiles (SLBMs), land based intercontinental ballistic missiles (ICBMs) and long-range bombers. (From:

参见“新战略三位一体”	Reference [72]) Refer to **“new strategic triad”**
局部战争【júbù zhànzhēng】	**local war**
聚变反应【jùbiàn fǎnyìng】	**fusion reaction**
聚变燃料【jùbiàn ránliào】	**fuel of fusion**
聚变威力【jùbiàn wēilì】	**fusion yield**
军备竞赛稳定性 【jūnbèi jìngsài wěndìngxìng】	**arms race stability**
军备控制【jūnbèi kòngzhì】	**arms control**
军事变革【jūnshì biàngé】 将先进的技术和武器系统，与创新的军事学说和组织体制结合在一起，使军事作战的特点和方式发生根本性的变化，军队的作战效能达到极大提高的根本性改革。(改自：参考文献[1]，p47)	**revolution in military affairs (RMA)** Fundamental reforms that thoroughly change the characteristics and patterns of military operations so as to greatly enhance operational effectiveness of the military through advanced technology and weapons systems combined with innovative military doctrines and organizational mechanisms. (Modified from: Reference [1], p47)
军事稳定性【jūnshì wěndìngxìng】	**military stability**
开放天空条约 【kāifàng tiānkōng tiáoyuē】	**Open Skies Treaty**
抗干扰【kàng gānrǎo】	**tamper resistance**
抗核加固【kànghé jiāgù】	**nuclear hardening**
科尔太克斯法【kē'ěrtàikèsī fǎ】 (连续反射法测量半径随时间变化的实验)	**CORRTEX (continuous reflectometry for radius vs time experiment)**
可裂变材料【kělièbiàn cáiliào】 一般而言，指能产生核裂变的一种同位素或同位素混合物。有些可裂变材料只有在足够快的中子(如动能超过 1 MeV 的中子)作用下才能	**fissionable material** In general, an isotope or a mixture of isotopes capable of nuclear fission. Some fissionable materials are capable of fission only by sufficiently fast neutrons (e.g. neutrons of a kinetic

汉—英

发生裂变。在所有能量的中子包括慢(热)中子作用下都可以发生裂变的同位素通常称之为易裂变材料或易裂变同位素。例如，同位素 铀-233，铀-235，钚-239，钚-241 既被称为可裂变材料又被称为易裂变材料，而铀-238 和钚-240 仅被称为可裂变材料而不是易裂变材料。(源自：参考文献[4]，4.6)	energy above 1 MeV). Isotopes that undergo fission by neutrons of all energies, including slow (thermal) neutrons, are usually referred to as fissile materials or fissile isotopes. For example, isotopes U-233, U-235, Pu-239 and Pu-241 are referred to as both fissionable and fissile, while U-236 and Pu-240 are fissionable but not fissile. (From: Reference[4], 4.6)
可区分性展示【kěqūfēnxìng zhǎnshì】	**distinguishability exhibition**
可疑场地视察【kěyí chǎngdì shìchá】	**suspect-site inspection**
可用于武器的材料【kěyòngyú wǔqì de cáiliào】	**weapon-usable material**
可转换材料【kězhuǎnhuàn cáiliào】通过在一个原子核中俘获一个中子而能被转化为特种可裂变材料的一种核材料。(源自：参考文献[4]，4.7)	**fertile material** Nuclear material that can be converted into a special fissionable material through capture of one neutron per nucleus. (From: Reference [4], 4.7)
空中核爆炸【kōngzhōng hébàozhà】	**nuclear airburst**
库存核武器可靠性【kùcún héwǔqì kěkàoxìng】	**reliability of stockpile nuclear weapon**
快堆【kuàiduī】	**fast reactor**
快中子【kuàizhōngzǐ】	**fast neutrons**
快中子临界装置【kuàizhōngzǐ línjiè zhuāngzhì】	**fast-neutron criticality facility**
快中子脉冲堆【kuàizhōngzǐ màichōng duī】	**fast-neutron pulse reactor**
亏量【kuīliàng】	**defect**
扩散分离机组【kuòsàn fēnlí jīzǔ】	**diffusion separation unit**
扩散分离器【kuòsàn fēnlíqì】	**diffuser**

拉丁美洲和加勒比海禁止核武器条约 【lādīngměizhōu hé jiālèbǐhǎi jìnzhǐ héwǔqì tiáoyuē】	**Treaty for the Prohibition of Nuclear Weapons in Latin America and the Caribbean**
滥用【lànyòng】	**misuse**
雷道克斯流程【léidàokèsī liúchéng】	**redox process**
累积辐照剂量【lěijī fúzhào jìliàng】	**cumulative radiation dose**
冷战【lěngzhàn】	**cold war**
离心分离工厂【líxīn fēnlí gōngchǎng】	**centrifuge separation plant**
离心机失效率【líxīnjī shīxiàolǜ】	**centrifuge failure rate**
离心机专用变频电源 【líxīnjī zhuānyòng biànpín diànyuán】	**variable frequency power for special purpose of a centrifuge**
离心机转子材料 【líxīnjī zhuànzǐ cáiliào】	**centrifuge rotor material**
离心机转子动力学 【líxīnjī zhuànzǐ dònglìxué】	**centrifuge rotor dynamics**
离心机阻尼装置 【líxīnjī zǔní zhuāngzhì】	**centrifuge damping device**
离子【lízǐ】	**ion**
锂【lǐ】	**lithium**
锂同位素分离【lǐ tóngwèisù fēnlí】	**lithium isotopes separation**
例行视察【lìxíng shìchá】	**routine inspection**
连续视察【liánxù shìchá】 为达到保障监督目的，通过察看关键操作、记录测量和运行的数据并核实这些信息，借以持续地掌握材料的库存清单和流向情况的视察机制。(源自：参考文献[4]，11.12)	**continuous inspection** An inspection regime intended to maintain continuity of knowledge concerning inventory and flow of nuclear material by witnessing key operations, recording measurement and operating data, and verifying the information in order to meet the safeguards objectives. (From: Reference [4], 11.12)
联大裁军特别会议 【liándà cáijūn tèbié huìyì】	**Special Session of the General Assembly Devoted to Disarmament**

联大裁军特别会议最后文件【liándà cáijūn tèbié huìyì zuìhòu wénjiàn】	**Final Document of the Special Session of the General Assembly Devoted to Disarmament**
联合国裁军审议委员会【liánhéguó cáijūn shěnyì wěiyuánhuì】	**United Nations Disarmament Commission (UNDC)**
联合国裁军事务部【liánhéguó cáijūn shìwùbù】	**United Nations Office (Department) for Disarmament Affairs**
联合国裁军事务咨询委员会【liánhéguó cáijūn shìwù zīxún wěiyuánhuì】	**United Nations Advisory Board on Disarmament Affairs**
联合国裁军研究所【liánhéguó cáijūn yánjiūsuǒ】	**United Nations Institute for Disarmament Research (UNIDIR)**
联合国常规军备委员会【liánhéguó chángguī jūnbèi wěiyuánhuì】	**United Nations Commission for Conventional Armaments**
联合国常规武器转让登记册【liánhéguó chángguī wǔqì zhuǎnràng dēngjìcè】	**United Nations Register of Conventional Weapons**
联合国大会【liánhéguó dàhuì】	**UN General Assembly**
联合国大会第一委员会【liánhéguó dàhuì dìyī wěiyuánhuì】	**First Committee of the UN General Assembly**
联合国关于侵略定义的决议【liánhéguó guānyú qīnlüè dìngyì de juéyì】	**UN resolution concerning the definition of aggression**
联合国宪章【liánhéguó xiànzhāng】	**United Nations Charter**
链式反应【liànshì fǎnyìng】	**chain reaction**
两面下注战略【liǎngmiàn xiàzhù zhànlüè】 尽可能促进和他国合作但也为敌对活动做准备的一种均衡做法。(改自：参考文献[45])	**hedging strategy** A balanced approach to foster cooperation with a nation where possible while also preparing for hostile activity. (Modified from: Reference [45])

裂变爆炸过早点火 【lièbiàn bàozhà guòzǎo diǎnhuǒ】	**predetonation in fission explosion**
裂变产额/裂变威力 【lièbiàn chǎn'é lièbiàn wēilì】	**fission yield**
裂变武器【lièbiàn wǔqì】	**fission weapon**
裂变中子【lièbiàn zhōngzǐ】	**fission neutrons**
临界安全评估【línjiè ānquán pínggū】 为确保核武器用的可裂变材料在生产、加工、运输及装配过程中均处于次临界安全状态所进行的实验和分析。(改自：参考文献[2]，p40)	**criticality safety assessment** Analyses and experiments made to ensure fissionable materials used for nuclear weapons remains in a subcritical and safe state during the whole process of production, processing, transportation and assembly. (Modified from: Reference [2], p40)
临界装置【línjiè zhuāngzhì】	**critical assembly**
临时通知视察【línshí tōngzhī shìchá】 IAEA 对一个国家的一处设施或设施外的一处场地进行视察时，提前通报时间比 INFIRCIR/153 协议的第 83 段规定的通报时间短的视察。(源自：参考文献[4]，11.7)	**short-notice inspection** An inspection performed at a facility or a location outside facilities for which less advance notice is provided by the IAEA to the State than that provided for under paragraph 83 of [IAEA INFIRCIR 153]. (From: Reference [4], 11.7)
灵活反应战略 【línghuó fǎnyìng zhànlüè】	**strategy of flexible response**
零威力实验【língwēilì shíyàn】 参见"次临界实验"	**zero-yield experiment** Refer to "**subcritical experiment**"
流体动力学实验 【liútǐ dònglìxué shíyàn】 为模拟核爆炸内爆过程所进行的实验。它是用代用材料(如铀-238、钨、钢等)替代核装置中的裂变材料高浓铀或钚-239、用高能炸药爆炸压缩该装置的整体或部分结构而进行	**hydrodynamic experiment** An experiment used to simulate the implosion process of a nuclear explosive. It uses other materials such as U-238, tungsten and steel as substitute for fissile materials such as HEU or Pu-239 in a nuclear device, and uses the high explosive to compress the

的一种实验。由于装置中的材料在高能炸药爆炸压缩下处于流体状态，因此称此类实验为流体动力学实验。这种实验没有核能释放，实验不一定要在核试验场地进行。(源自：参考文献[1]，p212-213)	whole or partial structure of the device. As the materials are in the liquid state under the compression of explosion of high explosive, such experiments are called hydrodynamic experiments. The experiment releases no nuclear energy and is not required to be conducted at a nuclear test site. (From: Reference [1], p212-213)
流体核实验【liútǐ héshíyàn】 一种评估核武器某些安全问题的方法，由洛斯·阿拉莫斯国家实验室(LANL)在 1958 年至 1961 年的暂停核试验期间研究核爆炸"一点安全"时首先使用。该实验在次临界增殖装置中或极轻微的超临界状态下进行，在某些情况下会释放小于 7 兆焦设计限额的裂变能。(改自：参考文献[30]，p1)	**hydronuclear experiment** A method for assessing some aspects of nuclear weapon safety, first conducted at Los Alamos during the 1958-61 moratorium on nuclear testing to investigate the "one-point" safety of a nuclear explosive. The experiments resulted in subcritical multiplying assemblies or a very slight degree of supercriticality and, in some cases, involved a fission energy release less than the design limit of 7 megajoules. (Modified from: Reference [30], p1)
六氟化铀【liùfúhuàyóu】	**uranium hexafluoride**
六氟化铀水解【liùfúhuàyóu shuǐjiě】	**uranium hexafluoride hydrolysis**
六氟化铀转化 【liùfúhuàyóu zhuǎnhuà】	**conversion of uranium hexafluoride**
绿盐【lǜyán】 绿色的 UF_4 晶体，是铀工艺中 UF_4 的俗称。UF_4 是生产核燃料的重要中间产品，用于制备六氟化铀(UF_6)和金属铀。(源自：参考文献[2]，p304)	**green salt** The popular name of green uranium tetrafluoride (UF_4) crystal. It is an important mid-point production in the process of producing uranium fuel. It can be used to produce uranium hexafluoride (UF_6) and uranium metal. (From: Reference [2], p304)
慢中子【màn zhōngzǐ】	**slow neutrons**

美朝框架协议 【měi cháo kuàngjià xiéyì】	**Agreed Framework Between the United States of American and the Democratic People's Republic of Korea**
美俄关于进一步削减和限制进攻性战略武器条约 【měi é guānyú jìnyībù xuējiǎn hé xiànzhì jìngōngxìng zhànlüè wǔqì tiáoyuē】	**Treaty Between the United States of America and the Russian Federation on Further Reduction and Limitation of Strategic Offensive Arms (START II)**
美俄削减进攻性战略武器条约(莫斯科条约) 【měi é xuējiǎn jìngōngxìng zhànlüè wǔqì tiáoyuē mòsīkē tiáoyuē】	**Treaty Between the United States of America and the Russian Federation On Strategic Offensive Reductions (Moscow/SORT)**
美国 **1978** 年核不扩散法 【měiguó 1978 nián hébùkuòsàn fǎ】 核不扩散法声明了美国的政策：(1) 寻求建立核设备、核材料和核技术的国际控制；(2) 提高美国作为核反应堆和核燃料供应国的可靠性；(3) 鼓励批准《不扩散核武器条约》；(4) 帮助其他国家核实和调整适当的能源生产技术。 (改自：参考文献[35])	**U.S. Nuclear Non-Proliferation Act of 1978** The Nuclear Non-Proliferation Act declares it United States policy: (1) to pursue the establishment of inter-national controls of nuclear equipment, material, and technology, (2) to enhance the reliability of the United States as a supplier of nuclear reactors and fuels, (3) to encourage ratification of the Treaty on the Non-Proliferation of Nuclear Weapons, and (4) to aid other nations in identification and adaptation of appropriate energy production technology. (Modified from: Reference [35])
美苏关于防止核战争协定 【měi sū guānyú fángzhǐ hézhànzhēng xiédìng】	**Agreement Between the United States of America and the Union of Soviet Socialist Republics on the Prevention of Nuclear War**
美苏关于减少爆发核战争危险的措施的协定 【měi sū guānyú jiǎnshǎo bàofā hézhànzhēng wēixiǎn de cuòshī de xiédìng】	**Agreement on Measures to Reduce the Risk of Outbreak of Nuclear War Between the United States of America and the Union of Soviet Socialist Republics**

美苏关于建立减少核危险中心的协定 【měi sū guānyú jiànlì jiǎnshǎo héwēixiǎn zhōngxīn de xiédìng】	**Agreement Between the United States of America and the Union of Soviet Socialist Republics on the Establishment of Nuclear Risk Reduction Centers**
美苏关于限制反弹道导弹系统条约(反导条约) 【měi sū guānyú xiànzhì fǎn dàndàodǎodàn xìtǒng tiáoyuē fǎndǎo tiáoyuē】	**Treaty Between the United States of America and the Union of Soviet Socialist Republics on the Limitation of Anti-ballistic Missile Systems (ABM Treaty)**
美苏关于消除两国中程及中短程导弹条约(中导条约) 【měi sū guānyú xiāochú liǎngguó zhōngchéng jí zhōngduǎnchéng dǎodàn tiáoyuē zhōngdǎo tiáoyuē】	**Treaty Between the United States of America and the Union of Soviet Socialist Republics on the Elimination of Their Intermediate-Range and Shorter-Range Missiles (INF Treaty)**
美苏关于削减和限制进攻性战略武器条约 【měi sū guānyú xuējiǎn hé xiànzhì jìngōngxìng zhànlüèwǔqì tiáoyuē】	**Treaty Between the United States of America and the Union of Soviet Socialist Republics on the Reduction and Limitation of Offensive Strategic Arms (START I)**
美苏关于削减和限制进攻性战略武器条约议定书 【měi sū guānyú xuējiǎn hé xiànzhì jìngōngxìng zhànlüèwǔqì tiáoyuē yìdìngshū】	**Protocol to the Treaty Between the United States of America and the Union of Soviet Socialist Republics on the Reduction and Limitation of Strategic Offensive Arms**
美苏和平利用地下核爆炸条约 【měi sū hépíng lìyòng dìxià hébàozhà tiáoyuē】	**Treaty Between the United States of America and the Union of Soviet Socialist Republics on Underground Nuclear Explosion for Peaceful Purposes (PNE)**
美苏限制地下核武器试验条约(限当量条约) 【měi sū xiànzhì dìxià héwǔqì shìyàn	**Treaty Between the United States of America and the Union of Soviet Socialist Republics on the Limitation of**

tiáoyuē xiàndāngliàng tiáoyuē】	**Underground Nuclear Weapon Tests (TTBT)**
美苏限制进攻性战略武器的某些措施的临时协定 【měi sū xiànzhì jìngōngxìng zhànlüè wǔqì de mǒuxiē cuòshī de línshí xiédìng】	**Interim Agreement Between the United States of America and the Union of Soviet Socialist Republics on Certain Measures with Respect to the Limitation of Strategic Offensive Arms (SALT I)**
美苏限制进攻性战略武器条约 【měi sū xiànzhì jìngōngxìng zhànlüè wǔqì tiáoyuē】	**Treaty Between the United States of America and the Union of Soviet Socialist Republics on the Limitation of Strategic Offensive Arms (SALT II Treaty)**
盟约【méngyuē】	**covenant**
密码锁(亦称启动连接装置) 【mìmǎsuǒ yìchēng qǐdòng liánjiē zhuāngzhì】 一种安装或附加在核武器系统上的装置，用于在输入预定的离散密码前，防止解除保险和(或)发射。(源自：参考文献[9]，p412) 参见“**核武器保险装置**”	**permissive action link (PAL)** A device included in or attached to a nuclear weapon system to preclude arming and/or launching until the insertion of a prescribed discrete code. (From: Reference[9], p412) Refer to “**safing device of nuclear weapon**”
面目标【miàn mùbiāo】	**area target**
模板法【móbǎnfǎ】 模板法是通过测量物体的某些特征，并与从某个参照物(如经认证的一件特定类型的武器)测得的同样一组特征(即模板)相比较。如果这两组数据测量相符，就可以判定该物体就是这种类型的武器。(源自：参考文献[11]，p99)	**template approach** The template approach to identify treaty-limited objects works by measuring certain characteristics of an object and comparing them with the same set of measurements taken from a reference object (e.g., an authentic weapon of a particular type): the template. (From: Reference [11],p99)
目标定位【mùbiāo dìngwèi】	**target positioning**

汉—英

目视观察【mùshì guānchá】	**visual observation**
内爆法原子弹 【nèibàofǎ yuánzǐdàn】	**implosion-type atomic bomb**
南太平洋无核区条约(拉罗汤加岛条约) 【nántàipíngyáng wúhéqū tiáoyuē lāluótāngjiādǎo tiáoyuē】	**South Pacific Nuclear Free Zone Treaty (Treaty of Rarotonga)**
逆流离心机【nìliú líxīnjī】	**countercurrent gas centrifuge**
逆流气体离心机的分离效率 【nìliú qìtǐ líxīnjī de fēnlí xiàolǜ】	**separation efficiency of a countercurrent gas centrifuge**
年(辐照)剂量【nián fúzhào jìliàng】	**annual dose**
年通过量【nián tōngguòliàng】	**annual throughput**
浓缩(富集)厂/同位素分离厂 【nóngsuō fùjí chǎng tóngwèisù fēnlíchǎng】	**enrichment plant/isotope separation plant**
浓缩(富集)度【nóngsuō fùjí dù】	**enrichment**
浓缩(富集)因子 【nóngsuō fùjí yīnzǐ】	**enrichment factor**
浓缩(富集)铀【nóngsuō fùjí yóu】	**enriched uranium**
欧洲安全与合作组织 【ōuzhōu ānquán yǔ hézuò zǔzhī】	**Organization for Security and Cooperation in Europe (OSCE)**
批数据【pīshùjù】	**batch data**
贫化【pínhuà】	**depletion**
贫化铀【pínhuàyóu】	**depleted uranium**
平洞地下核试验 【píngdòng dìxià héshìyàn】	**tunnel nuclear test**
破坏性分析【pòhuàixìng fēnxī】	**destructive analysis (DA)**
普雷克斯流程【pǔléikèsī liúchéng】 (钚铀的萃取回收流程)	**PUREX (Plutonium Uranium Recovery by Extraction) process**
谱分辨率【pǔ fēnbiànlǜ】	**spectral resolution**
起爆序列【qǐbào xùliè】	**initiating sequence**

起爆元件【qǐbào yuánjiàn】	**initiating component**
气体扩散的理想分离因子 【qìtǐ kuòsàn de lǐxiǎng fēnlí yīnzǐ】	**ideal separation factor of gaseous diffusion process**
气体扩散法【qìtǐ kuòsànfǎ】	**gaseous diffusion method**
气体扩散分离级的分离效率 【qìtǐ kuòsàn fēnlíjí de fēnlí xiàolǜ】	**stage separation efficiency of gaseous diffusion process**
气体扩散分离压缩机 【qìtǐ kuòsàn fēnlí yāsuōjī】	**compressor for gaseous diffusion separation**
气体扩散工厂 【qìtǐ kuòsàn gōngchǎng】	**gaseous diffusion plant**
气体离心机【qìtǐ líxīnjī】	**gas centrifuge**
气体离心机的供取料 【qìtǐ líxīnjī de gōngqǔliào】	**feed and withdrawals of a gas centrifuge**
气体离心机的最大理论分离功率 【qìtǐ líxīnjī de zuìdà lǐlùn fēnlí gōnglǜ】	**theoretical maximum separative power of a gas centrifuge**
气体离心机环流驱动法 【qìtǐ líxīnjī huánliú qūdòngfǎ】	**means to drive circulation in a gas centrifuge**
气体离心机流场【qìtǐ líxīnjī liúchǎng】	**flow field in gas centrifuge**
气体离心机转筒 【qìtǐ líxīnjī zhuàntǒng】	**rotor of a gas centrifuge**
前沿防御战略 【qiányán fángyù zhànlüè】	**forward defense strategy**
潜射弹道导弹 【qiánshè dàndàodǎodàn】	**submarine-launched ballistic missile**
枪法原子弹【qiāngfǎ yuánzǐdàn】	**gun-type atomic bomb**
切削(碎)料【qiēxuē suì liào】	**scrap**
切削(碎)料回收厂 【qiēxuē suì liào huíshōuchǎng】	**scrap recovery plant**
勤务保险【qínwù bǎoxiǎn】	**service safety**
氢弹【qīngdàn】	**hydrogen bomb**
氢弹构形【qīngdàn gòuxíng】	**configuration of hydrogen bomb**

氢化锂【qīnghuàlǐ】	**lithium hydride**
轻水堆【qīngshuǐduī】	**light water reactor (LWR)**
全面保障监督协定 【quánmiàn bǎozhàng jiāndū xiédìng】	**comprehensive (full scope) safeguards agreement (CSA)**
全面禁止核试验条约 【quánmiàn jìnzhǐ héshìyàn tiáoyuē】	**Comprehensive Test Ban Treaty (CTBT)**
全球战略【quánqiú zhànlüè】 泛指运用军事、经济、政治、外交等手段以实现和保护国家或国家集团在全球的利益的方略。(源自：参考文献[1]，p25)	**global strategy** Strategy that aims at achieving and maintaining global interests for a nation or a group of nations through military, economic, political, diplomatic and other means. (From: Reference [1], p25)
劝阻【quànzǔ】 在当前美国思维中，指劝说其他大国放弃与美国在军事能力方面的竞争。(源自：参考文献[41]) 注：在核学说范畴，法语单词“la dissuasion”实质上意指威慑。(源自：参考文献[69]，pII-41)	**dissuasion** In current U.S. thinking, “to persuade other powers to refrain from initiating a competition in military capabilities.” (From: Reference [41]) Note: In the context of nuclear doctrine, the French word, “la dissuasion” means essentially “deterrence”. (From: Reference [69], pII-41)
燃耗【ránhào】	**burnup**
燃料棒束【ránliàobàngshù】	**fuel bundle**
燃料部件【ránliào bùjiàn】	**fuel component**
燃料元件【ránliào yuánjiàn】	**fuel element**
燃料制造厂【ránliào zhìzàochǎng】	**fuel fabrication plant**
燃料组件【ránliào zǔjiàn】	**fuel assembly**
热核点火【rèhé diǎnhuǒ】	**thermonuclear ignition**
热核武器【rèhéwǔqì】	**thermonuclear weapon**
热室【rèshì】	**hot cell**

热中子【rèzhōngzǐ】	**thermal neutrons**
人工放射性核素 【réngōng fàngshèxìng hésù】	**artificial radionuclide**
熔盐电解精炼流程 【róngyán diànjiě jīngliàn liúchéng】	**molten salt electrorefining process**
弱冲击波聚焦【ruò chōngjībō jùjiāo】	**focusing of weak shock wave**
弱剩余放射性武器(3R 弹) 【ruò shèngyú fàngshèxìng wǔqì 3Rdàn】	**reduced residual radioactivity weapon (RRRW)**
三位一体战略核力量 【sānwèiyītǐ zhànlüè hélìliàng】 参见“旧核三位一体”	**triad strategic nuclear force** Refer to **“old nuclear triad”**
三相弹【sānxiàngdàn】 放能过程经历由裂变到聚变再到裂变三个阶段的一种氢弹，其最后的裂变阶段由临近于热核燃料的天然铀、贫铀或浓缩铀来完成。世界上大多数战略核武器都属于这种类型。(改自：参考文献[3]，p802)	**tri-phase bomb** A type of hydrogen bomb whose energy release process consists of three phases: fission, fusion, and then fission. The final fission phase is achieved by the use of natural uranium, depleted uranium, or enriched uranium in proximity to the thermonuclear fuel. Most strategic nuclear weapons in the world belong to this type. (Modified from: Reference [3], p802)
桑戈委员会【sānggē wěiyuánhuì】 一些有核出口能力的《不扩散核武器条约》(NPT)缔约国组成的核出口控制集团，又称 NPT 出口国委员会。该委员会于 1971 年成立，宗旨是控制《不扩散核武器条约》成员国对没有核武器的非条约成员国的核材料和核设备的出口，以防止核武器扩散。委员会的主要出口控制机制是“触发清单”，即向无核武	**Zangger Committee** The Zangger Committee, also known as the Nuclear Non-proliferation Treaty Exporters Committee, is a nuclear export group, which consists of parties of the Nuclear Non-proliferation Treaty (NPT) who have the capability of nuclear export. The committee was formed in 1971. It aims to prevent the prohibition of nuclear weapons by controlling the export of nuclear materials and equipment from parties of the NPT to non-nuclear-weapon states.

器国家出口触发清单上的项目，接收国必须接受“国际原子能机构”的保障监督。目前该委员会有 36 个成员国。(改自：参考文献[1]，p374)	The main export control mechanism of the committee is the “Trigger List”. Items on this List exported to non-nuclear- weapon states must be subject to IAEA safeguards. The committee now has 36 member states. (Modified from: Reference [1], p374)
桑戈委员会出口准则【sānggē wěiyuánhuì chūkǒu zhǔnzé】	**Zangger Committee Export Guidelines**
杀手锏【shāshǒujiǎn】 锏是一种由金属制成的冷兵器。在中国古典小说中指与敌厮杀时出其不意地用锏投掷敌手、以求取胜的招数。喻指在关键时刻使出的最拿手的本领或称绝招。(改自：参考文献[36])	**assassin's mace** A type of metal weapon. Chinese classical novels describe the means of throwing the mace at the adversary unexpectedly in order to win during fighting. It is a metaphor for an adept ability or unique skill used at a critical moment. (Modified from: Reference [36])
闪光 X 射线照相【shǎnguāng X shèxiàn zhàoxiàng】	**flash radiography by pulsed X-ray system**
嬗变【shànbiàn】	**transmutation**
设计资料核查【shèjì zīliào héchá】	**design information verification (DIV)**
设施关闭视察【shèshī guānbì shìchá】	**close-out inspection**
设施外场所【shèshīwài chǎngsuǒ】	**location outside facilities (LOF)**
设施周边与进出口连续监测【shèshī zhōubiān yǔ jìnchūkǒu liánxù jiāncè】	**perimeter portal continuous monitoring**
射程【shèchéng】	**firing range**
生产堆【shēngchǎnduī】	**production reactor**
声明【shēngmíng】	**statement**
湿法贮存【shīfǎ zhùcún】	**wet storage**
十八国裁军委员会【shíbāguó cáijūn wěiyuánhuì】	**Eighteen-Nation Committee on Disarmament (ENCD)**

十国裁军委员会 【shíguó cáijūn wěiyuánhuì】	**Ten-Nation Committee on Disarmament (TNCD)**
石墨慢化堆【shímò mànhuàduī】	**graphite moderated reactor**
时间分辨率 【shíjiān fēnbiànlǜ】	**temporal resolution**
实际级联【shíjì jílián】	**real cascade**
实时监测【shíshí jiāncè】 除了电子通信所必需的时间外，没有显著延迟地对数据或信息进行的及时的监测。(源自：参考文献[9]，p451)	**real-time monitoring** Monitoring information which has been delayed only by the time required for electronic communication, implying that there are no noticeable delays. (Modified from: Reference [9], p451)
实体保护建议【shítǐ bǎohù jiànyì】	**physical-protection recommendations**
实体保护控制中心 【shítǐ bǎohù kòngzhì zhōngxīn】	**control center for physical protection**
实体保护设计基准威胁 【shítǐ bǎohù shèjì jīzhǔn wēixié】	**physical-protection design basis threats**
实体保护探测系统 【shítǐ bǎohù tàncè xìtǒng】	**detection system for physical protection**
实体保护通信系统 【shítǐ bǎohù tōngxìn xìtǒng】	**communication system for physical protection**
实体保护系统失效判断准则 【shítǐ bǎohù xìtǒng shīxiào pànduàn zhǔnzé】	**physical-protection system-failure criterion**
实体保护应急响应 【shítǐ bǎohù yìngjí xiǎngyìng】	**physical-protection emergency response**
实体保护组织机构 【shítǐ bǎohù zǔzhī jīgòu】	**physical-protection organization**
实体(实物)保护报警系统 【shítǐ shíwù bǎohù bàojǐng xìtǒng】	**alarm system for physical protection**
实物存量【shíwù cúnliàng】 某一给定时刻，在特定核材料平衡区内，按照规定程序测量或估算所得到的所有批量的核材料总和。(改	**physical inventory** The sum of all the measured or derived estimates of batch quantities of nuclear material on hand at a given time within a material balance area, obtained in

汉-英

自：参考文献[15]，para113；[4]，6.41)	accordance with specified procedures. (Modified from: Reference [15], para113; [4], 6.41)
实战部署的弹头【shízhàn bùshǔ de dàntóu】	**operationally deployed warhead**
实战能力【shízhàn nénglì】	**operational capability**
手套箱【shǒutàoxiāng】	**glove box**
属性法【shǔxìngfǎ】 通过测量物项的某些特征来识别条约限定物项的方法。这些特征为某特定类型的所有物项所具备。(改自：参考文献[11]，p104)	**attribute approach** Identifies treaty-limited objects by measuring certain characteristics of an object that should be displayed by all items of a given general type. (Modified from: Reference [11], p104)
属性检验【shǔxìng jiǎnyàn】 判断一个物项的某项特征(或属性)为"是"或"否"的统计试验。(源自：参考文献[4]，10.30)	**attributes test** A statistical test of a characteristic (or attribute) of an item to which the response is either "yes" or "no". (From: Reference [4], 10.30)
竖井地下核试验【shùjǐng dìxià héshìyàn】	**shaft nuclear test**
数据更新视察【shùjù gēngxīn shìchá】	**data update inspection**
衰变【shuāibiàn】	**decay**
衰变能【shuāibiànnéng】	**decay energy**
双边合作协定【shuāngbiān hézuò xiédìng】	**bilateral cooperation agreement**
双循环流程【shuāngxúnhuán liúchéng】	**two cycle process**
水法后处理【shuǐfǎ hòuchǔlǐ】	**aqueous reprocessing**
水氟化流程【shuǐfúhuà liúchéng】	**aquafluor process**
水面及水下核爆炸毁伤效应【shuǐmiàn jí shuǐxià hébàozhà huǐshāng xiàoyìng】	**damaging and injuring effects of shallow or underwater nuclear explosion**
水声监测【shuǐshēng jiāncè】	**hydroacoustic monitoring**

四氟化铀氟化生产六氟化铀【sìfúhuàyóu fúhuà shēngchǎn liùfúhuàyóu】	**production of uranium hexafluoride by fluorination of uranium tetrafluoride**
随机取样【suíjī qǔyàng】 所涉群体内的所有物项有相同被选概率的取样方式。(源自：参考文献[4]，7.8)	**random sampling** The process of selecting samples in such a manner that all items in a population have the same probability of being selected. (From: Reference [4], 7.8)
随机视察【suíjī shìchá】 在一个随机选定的日期对一处设施或设施外的一处场地进行的视察。(源自：参考文献[4]，11.8)	**random inspection** An inspection performed at a facility or a location outside facilities on a date chosen randomly. (From: Reference [4], 11.8)
梭雷克斯流程【suōléikèsī liúchéng】(钍萃取流程)	**THOREX (thorium extraction) process**
探知概率【tànzhī gàilǜ】	**detection probability**
探知时间【tànzhī shíjiān】	**detection time**
特别视察【tèbié shìchá】	**ad hoc inspection**
特殊效应核武器【tèshū xiàoyìng héwǔqì】	**tailored effects nuclear weapon**
特种可裂变材料【tèzhǒng kělièbiàn cáiliào】 钚-239；铀-233；浓缩了同位素铀-235或铀-233的铀；任何含上述一种或多种物质的材料；以及IAEA理事会随时确定的其他可裂变材料；但“特种可裂变材料”不包括源材料。(源自：参考文献[4]，4.5)	**special fissionable material** Plutonium-239; uranium-233; uranium enriched in the isotopes 235 or 233; any material containing one or more of the foregoing; and such other fissionable material as the IAEA of Governors shall from time to time determine; but the term “special fissionable material” does not include source material. (From: Reference [4], 4.5)
梯恩梯当量【tī'ēntī dāngliàng】	**TNT equivalent**
天然放射性核素【tiānrán fàngshèxìng hésù】	**natural radionuclides**
天然铀【tiānrányóu】	**natural uranium**

停产的设施【tíngchǎn de shèshī】	**standby facility**
停堆换料动力堆 【tíngduī huànliào dònglìduī】	**off-load refuelled power reactor**
同时视察【tóngshí shìchá】 IAEA 视察员同时或在短时间内对一个国家的两处或多处设施进行视察，以发现设施之间可能进行的串通行为，例如设施之间相互临时转移(借用)核材料，从而使同一份核材料被 IAEA 核查两次，即在两个被视察的设施中各被核查一次。(源自：参考文献[4]，11.11)	**simultaneous inspections** Inspections performed by IAEA inspectors simultaneously or within a short period of time at two or more facilities in a State in order to detect possible diversions arranged in collusion between facilities by, for example, the temporary transfer ("borrowing") of nuclear material between facilities so that the same material would be verified twice by the IAEA, once in each of the two facilities inspected. (From: Reference [4], 11.11)
同位素【tóngwèisù】	**isotope**
同位素分离【tóngwèisù fēnlí】	**isotope separation**
同位素分离因子 【tóngwèisù fēnlí yīnzǐ】 表征分离单元分离效果的特征量，表示某一分离效应所产生同位素相对丰度的变化情况。(源自：参考文献[2]，p404)	**isotope separation factor** A characteristic value for measuring separative efficiency of a separative unit. It is the ratio of the relative concentration after and before processing. (From: Reference [2], p404)
同位素位移【tóngwèisù wèiyí】	**isotope shift**
透明度【tòumíngdù】 信息公开。在核查领域可指国家军事活动和可能带有军事意味的和平活动(如军民两用技术)的公开。(源自：参考文献[54])	**transparency** Openness of information. In the verification field it may refer to openness about a state's military activities and about any peaceful activities that may have military implications (such as dual-use technology). (From: Reference [54])

钍-铀核燃料循环 【tǔ yóu héránliào xúnhuán】	**thorium-uranium nuclear fuel cycle**
退役设施/退役的设施外场所 【tuìyì shèshī tuìyì de shèshīwài chǎngsuǒ】	**decommissioned facility/decommissioned location outside facilities**
外空军事化【wàikōng jūnshìhuà】 在外空部署设施(通常是卫星)为军事活动提供信息支持。(改自：参考文献[56]，p30) 参见“外空武器化”	**militarization of space** The deployment of assets (typically satellites) in space for providing information support to military activities. (Modified from: Reference [56], p30) Refer to “**weaponization of space**”
外空武器化【wàikōng wǔqìhuà】 部署专门设计用于在/从外空作战的系统或部件，或部署专门设计用于在地球上攻击外空中目标的军事能力。(改自：参考文献[56]，p29) 参见“外空军事化”	**weaponization of space** To deploy systems or components specifically designed to fight a war in or from space, or military capabilities on the earth specifically designed to destroy or disable targets in space. (Modified From: Reference [56], p29) Refer to “**militarization of space**”
万隆会议十项原则 【wànlóng huìyì shíxiàng yuánzé】	**Ten Principles of the Bandung Conference**
危机管理【wēijī guǎnlǐ】 控制和管理危机，使其不至于失控而导致战争的过程。危机管理应确保解决危机以保障国家攸关利益。(改自：参考文献[28]，p240)	**crisis management** Procedures for controlling and managing a crisis so that it does not get out of hand and lead to war. Crisis management also ensures that the crisis is resolved so that the vital interests of the states involved are secured and protected. (Modified from: Reference [28], p240)
危机控制【wēijī kòngzhì】 泛指遵循维护国家利益和避免武力冲突的原则而抑制危机扩展的一系列互动过程：在危机尚处潜在阶段时努力消除可能促其爆发的因素；	**crisis control** A series of interactive processes carried out following the principle of safeguarding national interests and avoiding armed conflicts, to eliminate the factors that may impel the eruption of latent crisis;

汉-英

在危机爆发时促其尽快向缓解方向转化，因势利导，尽可能降低对抗程度。(改自：参考文献[1]，p42)	to lessen the seriousness of the crisis as soon as possible, and to reduce the degree of rivalry and contain the expansion of the crisis. (Modified from: Reference [1], p42)
危机稳定性【wēijī wěndìngxìng】	**crisis stability**
威逼【wēibī】 威胁使用武力以迫使敌手采取己方期望的行动。(源自：参考文献[23]) 注：威逼致力于终止已发生的行为而威慑致力于防止未发生的行动。(源自：参考文献[39]) 衍生：威逼，通常包括发起(威胁性)的行动(或诉诸行动的不可更改的决心)，只有在对手作出(妥协性的)反应后才能终止或变得无害。(源自：参考文献[23])	**compellence** The use of the threat of force to compel a desired action by one's adversary. (From: Reference [23]) Note: compellence refers to efforts to stop an action already underway whereas deterrence refers to efforts to prevent future action. (From: Reference [39]) Derived from: "Compellence… usually involves initiating an action (or an irrevocable commitment to action) that can cease, or become harmless, only if the opponent responds." (From: Reference [23])
威力【wēilì】	**yield**
威慑【wēishè】 通过使对手害怕后果来防止其采取行动。威慑是一种由难以承受的反击行动所致的可信威胁的存在所引发的心理状态。(源自：参考文献[9]，p160) 参见"**威逼**"	**deterrence** The prevention from action by fear of the consequences. Deterrence is a state of mind brought about by the existence of a credible threat of unacceptable counteraction. (From: Reference [9], p160) Refer to "**compellence**"
微型中子源反应堆 【wēixíng zhōngzǐyuán fǎnyìngduī】	**miniature neutron source reactor (MNSR)**
未申报设施或设施外场所 【wèi shēnbào shèshī huò shèshīwài chǎngsuǒ】	**undeclared facility or location outside facilities (LOF)**

无核武器国家【wú héwǔqì guójiā】	**non-nuclear weapon state (NNWS)**
无源γ射线探测【wúyuán γ shèxiàn tàncè】 通过测量裂变材料衰变时产生的特征γ射线，对裂变材料及含裂变材料的装置进行快速、无损探测的方法。(源自：参考文献[1]，p495)	**passive gamma-ray detection** A rapid and non-destructive detection of fissionable materials and equipments containing fissionable material through detecting characteristic gamma-rays emitted from decay of such fissionable material. (From: Reference [1], p495)
无源标签【wúyuán biāoqiān】 参见"**标签**"	**passive tag** Refer to "**tag**"
无源封记【wúyuán fēngjì】 参见"**封记**"	**passive seal** Refer to "**seal**"
无源中子探测【wúyuán zhōngzǐ tàncè】 通过探测裂变材料的自发中子而对裂变材料或含裂变材料的装置进行快速无损探测的方法。(源自：参考文献[1]，p495)	**passive neutron detection** A method of rapid non-destructive detection of fissionable material or devices containing fissionable materials by detecting neutrons spontaneously emitted from such fissionable material. (From: Reference [1], p496)
武器化【wǔqìhuà】	**weaponization**
武器级钚【wǔqìjí bù】 含小于或等于 7%以下钚-240 的钚。(源自：参考文献[1]，p233) 注：含远大于 7%以上钚-240 的钚事实上亦可用于核武器。(源自：参考文献[13]，p32-33)	**weapon-grade plutonium** Plutonium containing no more than 7% Pu-240. (From: Reference [1], p233) Note: Pu containing much more than 7% Pu-240 can actually be used in a nuclear weapon. (From: Reference [13], p32-33)
武器级铀【wǔqìjí yóu】 含大于或等于 90%以上铀-235 的铀。(源自：参考文献[1]，p233)	**weapon-grade uranium** Enriched uranium containing no less than 90% U-235. (From: Reference [1], p233)
物件计数【wùjiàn jìshù】	**item counting**

物理包【wùlǐbāo】 核武器中封装在辐射壳内的初级和次级部件的完整的组装件。(源自：参考文献[11]，p91)	**physics package** The primary and secondary of a nuclear weapon are housed inside a radiation case; the completed assembly is called the "physics package." (From: Reference [11], p91)
误差【wùchā】	**error**
西方国家集团 【xīfāng guójiā jítuán】	**Western Group**
吸收【xīshōu】	**absorption**
吸收剂量【xīshōu jìliàng】	**absorbed dose**
系统电磁脉冲 【xìtǒng diàncí màichōng】	**system-generated electromagnetic pulse**
系统取样【xìtǒng qǔyàng】 在一个连续的过程中以重复的方式进行取样，如每隔 10 个物项取样或每隔一定的时间间隔取样。(源自：参考文献[4]，7.9)	**systematic sampling** The process of selecting samples in a repeated pattern, such as every 11th item or at fixed time intervals, from a continuing process. (From: Reference [4], 7.9)
下游设施【xiàyóu shèshī】	**downstream facility**
先发制人打击【xiānfāzhìrén dǎjī】	**preemptive strike**
先前申报设施视察 【xiānqián shēnbào shèshī shìchá】	**formerly declared facility inspection**
现场视察【xiànchǎng shìchá】 在被探测现场利用人员或仪器收集信息的视察方式。《美苏关于削减和限制进攻性战略武器条约》规定了 13 种现场视察方式。视察由指派的视察员执行，旨在核实没有进行军备限制协议所禁止的活动，确认执行了军备限制协议所规定的活动，或调查可疑事件的真相。(改自：	**on-site inspection (OSI)** The verification method carried out by personnel or apparatus on the selected site. The 13 types of inspection are defined in the START I treaty. Inspections are carried out by designated inspectors to verify that particular activities prohibited by an arms limitation agreement are not performed, to check that particular activities prescribed by an arms limitation agreement are implemented,

参考文献[16]，p231)	or to examine the nature of a suspicious event. (Modified from:Reference [16], p231)
现场视察中的地球物理勘测【xiànchǎng shìchá zhōng de dìqiú wùlǐ kāncè】	**geophysical survey in on-site inspections**
现实威慑战略【xiànshí wēishè zhànlüè】	**strategy of realistic deterrence**
现役弹头【xiànyì dàntóu】	**active warhead**
现役核武库【xiànyì héwǔkù】	**active nuclear stockpile**
限制【xiànzhì】	**limit**
限制准入【xiànzhì zhǔnrù】 指在被视察国的要求下，IAEA 和该国达成的限制进入权限的安排。这种安排应按照“防止与扩散相关的敏感信息的散布、满足安全或实体保护要求或者保护所有权或商业敏感信息”的原则制定。(源自：参考文献[4]，11.26)	**managed access** Upon the request of a State, the IAEA and the State shall make arrangements for managed access, arranged in such a way as “to prevent the dissemination of proliferation sensitive information, to meet safety or physical protection requirements, or to protect proprietary or commercially sensitive information.” (From: Reference [4], 11.26)
宪章【xiànzhāng】	**charter**
相互确保摧毁战略【xiānghù quèbǎocuīhuǐ zhànlüè】	**strategy of mutual assured destruction (MAD)**
响应力量【xiǎngyìng lìliàng】 意指在遭遇潜在的意外事故时能增加作战部署力量的能力。它使领导层能握有根据危机发展的程度而增加作战部署力量数量的选择权。(改自：参考文献[66])	**responsive force** The responsive force is intended to provide a capability to augment the operationally deployed force to meet potential contingencies. It retains the option for leadership to increase the number of operationally deployed forces in proportion to the severity of an evolving crisis. (Modified from: Reference [66])
项目和供应协定【xiàngmù hé gōngyìng xiédìng】	**project and supply agreement**
销毁【xiāohuǐ】	**destruction**

汉—英

销毁视察【xiāohuǐ shìchá】	**elimination inspection**
小数量议定书 【xiǎoshùliàng yìdìngshū】	**small quantities protocol (SQP)**
协定/协议【xiédìng xiéyì】	**agreement**
芯块【xīnkuài】	**pellet**
新三位一体【xīn sānwèiyītǐ】 参见"新战略三位一体"	**new triad** Refer to "**new strategic triad**"
新设施视察【xīn shèshī shìchá】	**new facility inspection**
新思维【xīnsīwéi】 1　20世纪80年代中期苏联领导人戈尔巴乔夫对当时世界的看法以及关于苏联外交政策的观点，主要内容为：(1)世界是一个多样性的统一体；(2)充分尊重各国人民按照自己的选择而生活并独立自主地解决自身的问题；(3)全人类的利益高于阶级利益；(4)核战争威胁着人类的生存与发展；(5)全人类普遍安全的唯一原则基础是尊重主权。(改自:参考文献[1]，p34；[64]) 2 该术语用以描述20世纪80年代中后期在戈尔巴乔夫总统领导下而发展的苏联外交政策思维的特性。新思维的主要观点包括：(1)资本主义和社会主义之间不是"零和"关系；(2)共同的人类利益高于阶级利益；(3)与美国的军事均衡对苏联的安全不是必需的，非攻击性的防御	**new thinking** 1 The former Soviet Union President Mikhail Gorbachev's enunciated opinion on the world situation and Soviet Union foreign policy in the 1980s. The main points are: (1) The world is a unity of diversity. (2) Respect the choices of style of life according to people in each country and of the ways of solving their own problems independently. (3) The interest of humanity has priority over that of a class. (4) Nuclear war is a threat to human life and development. And (5) The basis of human common security is respect for independence and sovereignty of other members of the world community. (Modified From: Reference [1], p34; [64]) 2 The term used to characterize distinctive elements in Soviet foreign policy thinking developed under the leadership of President Mikhail Gorbachev in the latter half of the 1980s. The main propositions in new thinking included: (1) the relationship between capitalist and socialist states was not zero-sum; (2) common human interests should take priority over

战略应优于进攻战略；(4)军事力量主要用于防止冲突，而不是在战争中打败对手。新思维的某些表现形式包括单边裁军措施、削减军事力量、承诺单边和多边的信任建立及裁军措施。(源自：参考文献[57]，p117-129；[58])	class-based interests; (3) military parity with the U.S. was not necessary for Soviet security, and non-offensive defensive strategies were preferable to offensive strategies; (4) the main purpose of military power was to prevent conflict, rather than to defeat an adversary in a war. Some of the manifestations of new thinking included certain unilateral disarmament measures, reductions in the size of certain military forces, and a strong commitment to bilateral and multilateral confidence building and arms control measures. (From: Reference [57],p117-129; [58])
新战略三位一体 **【xīn zhànlüè sānwèiyītǐ】** 美国2002年《核态势评估》报告中提出的一种新的军事战略，由三部分组成：核与非核打击力量；主动的和被动的防御；全新的防御基础设施。(源自：参考文献[67]) 参见“**旧核三位一体**”	**new strategic triad** A new U.S. military strategy revealed in the 2002 Nuclear Posture Review, consisting of nuclear and non-nuclear strike forces; passive and active defenses; and a revitalized defense infrastructure. (From: Reference [67]) Refer to “**old nuclear triad**”
信息屏障【xìnxī píngzhàng】 用来保护鉴别过程中可能搜集到的敏感武器设计信息。这可以通过自动进行采集、储存和分析数据，并只向视察员提供分析的结果来实现。(改自：参考文献[11]，p107-108)	**information barrier** Used to protect any sensitive weapon design information that may be gathered during the identification process, for example, by automating the collection, storage, and analysis of data, and by making only the conclusions of the analysis available to the inspector. (Modified from: Reference [11], p107-108)
信息战【xìnxīzhàn】	**information warfare (IW)**
虚警率【xūjǐnglǜ】 被非真实事件驱动的报警次数与监	**false-alarm rate** The ratio of alarms triggered by real

测系统设计上所能侦测到的总报警次数的比例。虚警的产生是由于监测系统无法区分真实的或虚假的警报。(改自：参考文献[1]，p489)	events to the total number of alarms the monitoring system detects. The false alarms are generated because the monitoring system could not distinguish real from false alarms. (Modified from: Reference [1], p489)
虚拟核试验【xū'nǐ héshìyàn】 用先进的计算机程序和高性能计算机对核爆试验进行数值模拟。(改自：参考文献[2]，p430)	**virtual nuclear test** The numerical simulation of a nuclear explosion test done by advanced computer programs and high performance computers. (Modified from: Reference [2], p430)
宣言【xuānyán】	**declaration**
削减【xuējiǎn】	**reduction**
巡航导弹【xúnháng dǎodàn】	**cruise missile**
压水堆【yāshuǐduī】	**pressurized water reactor (PWR)**
亚临界气体离心机【yàlínjiè qìtǐ líxīnjī】	**subcritical gas centrifuge**
延伸(扩展)核威慑 【yánshēn kuòzhǎn héwēishè】 1 通过用核报复导致无法承受的毁伤以威胁觉察到的或潜在的敌手，防止其对盟国进行核打击的战略。 2 以威胁核报复来防止对其或其盟友进行常规打击的战略。(改自：参考文献[7]，p14-15)	**extended nuclear deterrence** 1 Strategy of preventing nuclear attack on one's allies by threatening the perceived or potential enemy with unacceptable damage by nuclear retaliation. 2 Strategy of preventing conventional attack on oneself or one's allies by threat of nuclear retaliation. (Modified from: Reference [7], p14-15)
研究堆【yánjiūduī】	**research reactor**
演习后疏散视察 【yǎnxíhòu shūsàn shìchá】	**post-exercise dispersal inspection**
验证与确认【yànzhèng yǔ quèrèn】 验证：是一个确定过程，即验证计算程序正确地求解了数学方程的过	**verification and validation (V&V)** Verification is the process of confirming that a computer code correctly

程。 确认：也是一个确定过程，即确认计算程序的计算结果恰当地描述了相关物理现象的过程。(改自：参考文献[63])	implements the algorithms that were intended. Validation is the process of confirming that the predictions of a code adequately represent measured physical phenomena. (Modified from: Reference [63])
样品【yàngpǐn】	**sample**
样品量【yàngpǐnliàng】	**sample size**
遥测数据打包和加密 【yáocè shùjù dǎbāo hé jiāmì】	**telemetry data packet and encryption**
遥感技术【yáogǎn jìshù】 用传感器远距离探测与条约有关的物项和(或)活动的技术。(改自：参考文献[19]，p235)	**remote sensing technology** Technology for detecting objects and/or activities at a distance by means of sensors. (Modified from: Reference [19], p235)
一次通过式核燃料循环 【yīcì tōngguòshì héránliào xúnhuán】	**once-through nuclear fuel cycle**
一体化保障监督 【yītǐhuà bǎozhàng jiāndū】 在全面保障监督协议及附加议定书下，国际原子能机构所能获得的所有保障监督手段的最佳组合，其目的是利用可拥有的资源，最有效、最高效地满足国际原子能机构规定的保障监督义务。(源自：参考文献[4]，3.5)	**integrated safeguards** The optimum combination of all safeguards measures available to the IAEA under comprehensive safeguards agreements and additional protocols to achieve maximum effectiveness and efficiency in meeting the IAEA's safeguards obligations within available resources. (From: Reference [4], 3.5)
一体化流程【yītǐhuà liúchéng】	**integral process**
已关闭设施/已关闭的设施外场所 【yǐguānbì shèshī yǐguānbì de shèshīwài chǎngsuǒ】	**closed-down facility/closed-down location outside facilities**
议定书【yìdìngshū】	**protocol**
易裂变材料 【yìlièbiàn cáiliào】	**fissile material**

易损性评定【yìsǔnxìng píngdìng】	**vulnerability assessment**
引控系统联试【yǐnkòng xìtǒng liánshì】	**integrated test of Arming, Fuzing & Firing (AF&F) system**
铀【yóu】	**uranium**
铀-233【yóu 233】	**uranium-233**
铀钚分离循环【yóu bù fēnlí xúnhuán】	**uranium-plutonium partition cycle**
铀钚混合氧化物【yóu bù hùnhé yǎnghuàwù】	**uranium-plutonium mixed dioxide**
铀钚循环【yóu bù xúnhuán】	**uranium-plutonium cycle**
铀产品的转化【yóuchǎnpǐn de zhuǎnhuà】	**conversion of uranium product**
铀纯化厂【yóu chúnhuàchǎng】	**uranium purification plant**
铀的氟化物【yóu de fúhuàwù】	**fluorides of uranium**
铀的中间氟化物【yóu de zhōngjiān fúhuàwù】	**intermediate fluorides of uranium**
铀光谱【yóu guāngpǔ】	**uranium spectrum**
铀合金【yóu héjīn】	**uranium alloy**
铀化学浓缩物【yóu huàxué nóngsuōwù】	**uranium chemical concentrate**
铀净化循环【yóu jìnghuà xúnhuán】	**uranium decontamination cycle**
铀矿开采和水冶【yóukuàng kāicǎi hé shuǐyě】	**uranium mine and ore processing**
铀同位素分离【yóu tóngwèisù fēnlí】	**uranium isotope separation**
铀氧化物的氟化【yóuyǎnghuàwù de fúhuà】	**fluorination of uranium oxide**
铀再循环【yóu zàixúnhuán】 将从乏燃料中回收得到的铀在反应堆内再循环使用的过程。(源自：参考文献[2]，p457)	**uranium recycling** A process of reusing the uranium extracted from spent fuel in nuclear reactors. (From: Reference [2], p457)

有关保障监督的修订补充协定 【yǒuguān bǎozhàng jiāndū de xiūdìng bǔchōng xiédìng】	**revised supplementary agreement relevant to safeguards**
有界波型电磁脉冲模拟器 【yǒujiè bōxíng diàncí màichōng mónǐqì】	**electromagnetic-pulse boundary-wave type simulator**
有限威慑【yǒuxiàn wēishè】 某些学者用于描述某种威慑形式所用的术语，但目前尚无定论。 注 1：在有些描述中，有限威慑要求有一定的核战能力，能够在核战争中的各升级阶梯上给对手造成损失，从而挫败对手使之不能取胜。(改自：参考文献[46]) 注 2：在有些描述中是指法国的核威慑。(改自：参考文献[18]，p360；[70]，p195-196) 注 3：“威慑”亦适应于非核情况。	**limited deterrence** A term used by some scholars to describe a form of deterrence. However, there is no consensus on the definition. Note 1：In some descriptions limited deterrence requires a limited warfighting capability to inflict costly damage on the adversary at every rung on the escalation ladder, thus denying the adversary victory in a nuclear war. (Modified from: Reference [46]) Note 2: In some descriptions it refers to France's nuclear deterrent. (Modified from: Reference [18], p360; [70], p195-196) Note 3: “deterrence” can also apply in non-nuclear circumstances.
有限战争【yǒuxiàn zhànzhēng】	**limited war**
有效载荷【yǒuxiào zàihè】	**payload**
有源标签【yǒuyuán biāoqiān】 参见“标签”	**active tag** Refer to “**tag**”
有源封记【yǒuyuán fēngjì】 参见“封记”	**active seal** Refer to “**seal**”
有源中子探测 【yǒuyuán zhōngzǐ tàncè】 利用外源诱发裂变材料裂变，通过探测裂变发出的中子而证实裂变材料存在的方法。(源自：参考文献[1]，p495)	**active neutron detection** A method of determining the existence of fissionable material through detecting the neutrons emitted from the fission that is induced by an external source. (From: Reference [1], p495)

余震监测【yúzhèn jiāncè】	**aftershock detection**
预警即发射【yùjǐng jì fāshè】	**launch-on-warning (LOW)**
预警卫星【yùjǐng wèixīng】	**early-warning satellite**
遇袭即发射【yùxí jì fāshè】	**launch-under-attack (LUA)**
原始数据【yuánshǐ shùjù】	**source data**
原子弹【yuánzǐdàn】	**atomic bomb**
原子弹弹芯【yuánzǐdàn dànxīn】 参见“弹芯”	**core of atomic bomb** Refer to “**pit**”
原子弹反射层(惰层) 【yuánzǐdàn fǎnshècéng duòcéng】	**reflector (tamper) layer in atomic bomb**
原子核【yuánzǐhé】	**atomic nucleus**
原子量【yuánzǐliàng】	**atomic mass**
原子能委员会 【yuánzǐnéng wěiyuánhuì】	**Atomic Energy Commission**
原子序数【yuánzǐ xùshù】	**atomic number**
原子蒸气激光同位素分离法 【yuánzǐ zhēngqì jīguāng tóngwèisù fēnlífǎ】	**atomic-vapor laser isotope separation**
圆概率偏差【yuán gàilǜ piānchā】 对于射弹、导弹或炸弹而言，其圆概率偏差是指，在反复试验中，包含其半数弹着点的圆形区域的半径。(改自：参考文献[9])	**circular error probable (CEP)** For repeated trials, the radius of a circle enclosing half of the impacts of a projectile, missile, or bomb. (Modified from: Reference [9])
源材料【yuáncáiliào】 含有天然形成的同位素混合体的铀；铀-235 被贫化的铀；钍；金属、合金、化合物或浓缩物状态的上述任何材料；任何含有一种或多种上述的物质并达到 IAEA 理事会随时确定的浓度的材料；以及理事会可	**source material** Uranium containing the mixture of isotopes occurring in nature; uranium depleted in the isotope 235; thorium; any of the foregoing in the form of metal, alloy, chemical compound, or concentrate; any other material containing one or more of the foregoing in such concentration as the IAEA Board of Governors shall from time to

随时确定的此类其他材料。根据[INFIRCIR/153]保障协定的 112 段：“源材料这一名词不适用于矿石或矿渣。”(源自：参考文献[4]，4.4)	time determine; and such other material as the Board of Governors shall from time to time determine. According to paragraph 112 of [IAEA INFCIRC/153], “the term source material shall not be interpreted as applying to ore or ore residue.” (From: Reference [4], 4.4)
运行记录【yùnxíng jìlù】	**operating records**
再入段【zàirùduàn】	**reentry phase**
暂停核试验【zàntíng héshìyàn】	**moratorium on nuclear testing**
暂停实施议定书 【zàntíng shíshī yìdìngshū】	**suspension protocol**
脏弹【zāngdàn】 参见“**放射性物质散布装置**”	**dirty bomb** Refer to “**radiological dispersal device (RDD)**”
增强 X 射线弹 【zēngqiáng X shèxiàndàn】	**enhanced X-ray weapon**
战略导弹【zhànlüè dǎodàn】	**strategic missile**
战略防御【zhànlüè fángyù】 1 战争全局上对进攻之敌的防御。它是战争中战略行动的基本类型之一，往往成为战争进程的一个阶段。战略防御的目的是阻止和挫败敌人的战略进攻，保存和积蓄自己的力量，消耗和消灭敌人，改变战场形势和力量对比，为转入战略进攻创造条件。(源自：参考文献[18]，p219) 2 挫伤敌人使用战略军事设施(主要是远程核运载系统)的能力。(改自：参考文献[71])	**strategic defense** 1 The defense against an offensive enemy in the overall situation of war. It is one of the basic types of strategic operations and usually becomes a stage in the course of war. The aim of strategic defense is to prevent and frustrate the enemy's strategic offense, preserve and save one's own strength, wear down and wipe out the enemy, change the battle situation and relative strength, and create conditions for shifting to strategic offense. (From: Reference [18], p219) 2 The capability to defeat an enemy's use of its strategic military assets, primarily long-range nuclear delivery systems. (Modified from: Reference [71])

战略防御倡议 【zhànlüè fángyù chàngyì】 罗纳德·里根总统在 1983 年 3 月 23 日声明的《战略防御倡议》指为拦截苏联射向美国的大规模战略导弹力量而建立的天基弹道导弹防御系统研制计划，俗称“星球大战”计划。(改自：参考文献[1]，p274；[17])	**strategic defense initiative (SDI)** The plan for a space-based ballistic missile defense system announced by U.S. president Ronald Reagan on March 23, 1983, aimed at defending against a mass attack of strategic nuclear missiles from the Soviet Union. It is also commonly called “Star Wars”. (Modified from: Reference [1], p274；[17])
战略核武器【zhànlüè héwǔqì】 1 用于打击战略目标，执行战略任务的核武器。(改自：参考文献[3],p1105) 2 战略核武器是指能打击远距离地域的战略目标(超过 5 500 公里)完成战略任务的武器。特殊情况下战略核武器可用于完成战役任务。战略核武器服役于战略核部队。(源自：参考文献[5]，p24) 注：战略担负对敌方及其军事力量产生长期的而非短期影响的使命。(改自：参考文献[9]，p516-517) 参见“**战术核武器**”	**strategic nuclear weapon** 1 Nuclear weapons that are used to strike strategic targets for strategic missions. (Modified from: Reference [3], p1105) 2 Strategic nuclear weapons are designed to engage objects in geographically remote strategic regions (over 5 500 km) to accomplish strategic missions. In exceptional situations, strategic nuclear weapons may be used to accomplish campaign missions. Strategic nuclear weapons are in service with the strategic nuclear forces. (From: Reference [5], p24) Note: Strategic refers to missions designed to have a long-term rather than immediate effect on the enemy and its military forces. (Modified from: Reference [9], p516-517) Refer to “**tactical nuclear weapon**”
战略稳定性【zhànlüè wěndìngxìng】	**strategic stability**
战略要点【zhànlüè yàodiǎn】	**strategic point**
战区核武器【zhànqū héwǔqì】	**theater nuclear weapon**
战术导弹【zhànshù dǎodàn】	**tactical missile**
战术核武器【zhànshù héwǔqì】 1 用于打击战役、战术纵深内重要	**tactical nuclear weapon** 1 Nuclear weapons used to attack in-depth key targets at the campaign

目标的核武器。(改自：参考文献[3]，p1107) 2　用于战场作战的核武器，诸如核炮弹、核炸弹和短程核导弹等。(改自：参考文献[8]) 3　战术核武器是指能打击敌方部署的战术纵深目标(最远 300 公里)完成战术任务的武器。在某些情况下，战术核武器可用于作战和战略任务，战略核炸弹也可用于战术目的。(改自：参考文献[5]，p24) 注 1：战术层面的活动是为完成战斗目的而关注涉及己方和敌方的作战要素的部署和调遣。(改自：参考文献[9]，p532) 注 2：战役是指军团为达成战争的局部目的或全局性目的，在统一指挥下进行的由一系列战斗组成的作战行动。(源自：参考文献[33]，p9) 参见“**战略核武器**”	and tactical level. (Modified from: Reference [3], p1107) 2 Nuclear weapons, such as artillery shells, bombs, and short-range missiles, for use in battlefield operations. (Modified from: Reference [8]) 3 Tactical nuclear weapons are designed to engage objects in the tactical depth of enemy deployment (up to 300 km) to accomplish a tactical mission. Under certain conditions, tactical nuclear weapons may be involved in operational and strategic missions. A strategic bomb can be used for tactical purposes. (Modified from: Reference [5], p24) Note 1: Activities at a tactical level focus on the ordered arrangement and maneuver of combat elements in relation to each other and to the enemy to achieve combat objectives. (Modified from: Reference [9], p532) Note 2: A campaign is a series of combat operations carried out by corps-level military forces under uniformed command to achieve partial or overall objectives. (From: Reference [33], p9) Refer to “**strategic nuclear weapon**”
账面平衡【zhàngmiàn pínghéng】	**account balance**
照射【zhàoshè】	**exposure**
针对性威慑【zhēnduìxìng wēishè】 根据目标国具体的心理、政治、意识形态，及经济状况而特别制订的灵活的威摄能力与实战原则。(源自：参考文献[21]，p49-51)	**tailored deterrence** Flexible deterrence capabilities and operational doctrines specifically designed according to the specific psychological, political, ideological, and economic characteristics of the targeted actor. (From: Reference[21], p49-51)

真实性验证 【zhēnshíxìng yànzhèng】	**authentication**
直接使用材料【zhíjiē shǐyòng cáiliào】 未经嬗变或进一步浓缩就可用于制造核爆炸装置的核材料。(源自：参考文献[4]，4.25)	**direct-use material** Nuclear material that can be used for the manufacture of nuclear explosive devices without transmutation or further enrichment. (From: Reference [4], 4.25)
指挥、控制、通信、计算和情报系统(C4I 系统) 【zhǐhuī kòngzhì tōngxìn jìsuàn hé qíngbào xìtǒng C4I xìtǒng】	**command, control,communications, computing and intelligence (C4I)**
指挥、控制、通信和情报系统(C3I 系统) 【zhǐhuī kòngzhì tōngxìn hé qíngbào xìtǒng C3I xìtǒng】	**command, control,communication and intelligence system (C3I)**
质子【zhìzǐ】	**proton**
滞留量【zhìliúliàng】	**hold-up**
中放废物【zhōngfàng fèiwù】	**intermediate-level radioactive waste**
中国防扩散出口管制体系 【zhōngguó fángkuòsàn chūkǒu guǎnzhì tǐxì】 中国关于核、生物、化学和导弹等各类敏感物项和技术及所有军品的全面的出口控制体制。(源自：参考文献[38])	**China's nonproliferation export control system** China's comprehensive export control system regarding various nuclear, biological, chemical and missile-related sensitive items, technology and all military goods. (From: Reference [38])
中国核出口三项原则 【zhōngguó héchūkǒu sānxiàng yuánzé】 中国核出口三项原则：第一，只用于和平目的；第二，接受国际原子能机构的保障和监督；第三，未经中国同意，接受国不得转让给第三国。(源自：参考文献[1]，p414)	**Three Principles on Nuclear Export Control of China** China's three principles of nuclear exports: guarantee for peaceful purposes only; acceptance of IAEA safeguards; and no retransfer to any third party without prior approval of the Chinese side. (From: Reference [1], p414)
中华人民共和国核出口管制条例 【zhōnghuá rénmín gònghéguó	**Regulations of the People's Republic of China on Nuclear**

hé chūkǒu guǎnzhì tiáolì】 中国政府于 1997 年 9 月 10 日公布《中华人民共和国核出口管制条例》，并宣布立即生效。条例共 22 条。(源自：参考文献[1]，p414) 注：该条例在 2006 年被修订了[74]。	**Export Control** The chinese government promulgated the Regulations of the People's Republic of China on Nuclear Export Control of on Sep.10, 1997, and declared that it took effect immediately. It has 22 articles. (From: Reference [1], p414) Note: this set of regulations was revised in 2006[74].
中华人民共和国核两用品及相关技术出口管制条例 【zhōnghuá rénmín gònghéguó hé liǎngyòngpǐn jí xiāngguān jìshù chūkǒu guǎnzhì tiáolì】 中国政府于 1998 年 6 月 10 日公布《中华人民共和国核两用品及相关技术出口管制条例》，条例从公布之日起生效。条例由 23 条正文和附件《核两用品及相关技术管制清单》组成。(源自：参考文献[1]，p415) 注：该条例在 2007 年被修订了[73]。	**Regulations of the People's Republic of China on Export Control of Dual-Use Nuclear Goods and the Related Technologies** The chinese government promulgated the Regulations of the People's Republic of China on Export Control of Dual-use Nuclear Goods and the Related Technologies on June 10, 1998. The Regulations took effect as of the date of promulgation. They consist of 23 articles and the Annex named the Nuclear Dual-Use Items and Related Technologies Export Control List. (From: Reference [1], p415) Note: this set of regulations was revised in 2007[73].
中华人民共和国主席和俄罗斯联邦总统关于互不首先使用核武器和互不将战略核武器瞄准对方的联合声明 【zhōnghuá rénmín gònghéguó zhǔxí hé éluósī liánbāng zǒngtǒng guānyú hùbù shǒuxiān shǐyòng héwǔqì hé hùbù jiāng zhànlüèhéwǔqì miáozhǔn duìfāng de liánhé shēngmíng】	**Joint Statement by the President of the People's Republic of China and the President of the Russian Federation on No-First-Use of Nuclear Weapons and Detargeting of Strategic Nuclear Weapons Against Each Other**
中间产品【zhōngjiān chǎnpǐn】	**intermediate product**
中子【zhōngzǐ】	**neutrons**
中子弹/增强辐射武器 【zhōngzǐdàn zēngqiáng fúshèwǔqì】	**neutron bomb/enhanced radiation weapon**

以高能中子为主要毁伤因素，相对减弱冲击波和光辐射效应的一种特殊设计的低威力氢弹。其较确切的名称是增强辐射武器。(改自：参考文献[1]，p152)	A low-yield hydrogen bomb with a special design utilizing high-energy neutrons as its main destructive element and relatively reducing its shock wave and thermal radiation effects. In a more accurate sense, it is called an "enhanced radiation weapon". (Modified from: Reference [1], p152)
重量分析【zhòngliàng fēnxī】	**gravimetric analysis**
重水【zhòngshuǐ】	**heavy water**
重水堆【zhòngshuǐduī】	**heavy water reactor (HWR)**
重水生产厂 【zhòngshuǐ shēngchǎnchǎng】	**heavy water production plant**
重要核设施【zhòngyào héshèshī】	**principal nuclear facility**
重要量【zhòngyàoliàng】 不能排除制造一枚核爆炸装置可能性的核材料的大致数量。(源自：参考文献[4]，3.14)	**significant quantity (SQ)** The approximate amount of nuclear material for which the possibility of manufacturing a nuclear explosive device cannot be excluded. (From: Reference [4], 3.14)
重要设备清单 【zhòngyào shèbèi qīngdān】	**essential equipment list (EEL)**
重铀酸铵【zhòngyóusuān'ān】	**ammonium diuranate**
逐步升级论【zhúbù shēngjílùn】	**theory of escalation**
主动段【zhǔdòngduàn】	**powered phase**
助爆型原子弹 【zhùbàoxíng yuánzǐdàn】	**boosted atomic bomb**
贮存设施【zhùcún shèshī】	**storage facility**
专门视察【zhuānmén shìchá】 一种在以下情况下进行的、被认为是很特殊的视察：在 INFIRCIR/153 协议中第 78-82 段规定的常规视察要求之外进行的视察；或者是想通	**special inspection** An inspection is deemed to be special: when it either is additional to the routine inspection effort provided for in paragraphs 78–82 of [IAEA INFCIRC/153], or involves access to information or locations in addition to

过获取或进入除 INFIRCIR/153 协议中第 76 段特别指明的可以进入的信息或场地之外的信息或场地进行的特别的和常规的视察；或者以上两种情况都包括的视察。(源自：参考文献[4] 11.13；[15])	the access specified in paragraph 76 of [IAEA INFCIRC/153] for ad hoc and routine inspections, or both. (From: Reference [4], 11.13; [15])
转化厂【zhuǎnhuàchǎng】	**conversion plant**
转化时间【zhuǎnhuà shíjiān】 将不同形式的核材料转化成核爆炸装置金属部件所需要的时间。(源自：参考文献[4]，3.13)	**conversion time** The time required to convert different forms of nuclear material to the metallic components of a nuclear explosive device. (From: Reference [4], 3.13)
转化视察【zhuǎnhuà shìchá】	**conversion inspection**
转让准则【zhuǎnràng zhǔnzé】	**transfer guideline**
转用策略/转用途径 【zhuǎnyòng cèlüè zhuǎnyòng tújìng】 一种(假定的)策略，即某国可能考虑转用国际原子能机构保障监督的核材料或不正当使用国际原子能机构保障监督的物项。转用策略可能包括：从一个受保障监督的设施内擅自转移核材料或利用一个受保障监督的核设施引进、生产或处理未申报的核材料。(源自：参考文献[4]，3.7)	**diversion strategy/diversion path** A (hypothetical) scheme which a State could consider to divert nuclear material or to misuse items subject to IAEA safeguards. Diversion strategies would include: the undeclared removal of nuclear material from a safeguarded facility or the use of a safeguarded facility for the introduction, production or processing of undeclared nuclear material. (From: Reference [4], 3.7)
自持热核燃烧【zìchí rèhé ránshāo】	**self-sustaining thermonuclear burn**
自发裂变【zìfā lièbiàn】	**spontaneous fission**
自卫防御核战略 【zìwèi fángyù hézhànlüè】 中国官方描述其核战略所用的术语。该战略的根本目标是遏制他国	**self-defensive nuclear strategy** Term used officially by China to describe its nuclear strategy. The strategy takes as its fundamental goal deterring other countries from using or

对中国使用或威胁使用核武器。该战略正式承诺在任何时候、任何情况下都不首先使用核武器的政策，无条件地承诺不对无核国家和无核地区使用或威胁使用核武器，主张全面禁止和彻底销毁核武器。该战略坚持自卫反击和有限发展的原则，着眼于建设一支满足国家安全需要的精干有效的核力量，确保核武器的安全性、可靠性，保持核力量的战略威慑作用。(改自：参考文献[34])	threatening to use nuclear weapons against China. It includes an official commitment to a policy of no first use of nuclear weapons at any time and under any circumstances. It unconditionally undertakes not to use or threaten to use nuclear weapons against non-nuclear-weapon states or nuclear-weapon-free zones, and stands for the comprehensive prohibition and complete elimination of nuclear weapons. The strategy upholds the principles of counterattack in self-defense and limited development of nuclear weapons, and aims at building a lean and effective nuclear force capable of meeting national security needs. It endeavors to ensure the security and reliability of its nuclear weapons and maintains a credible nuclear deterrent force. (Modified from: Reference [34])
自卫核反击【zìwèi héfǎnjī】 在遭受第一次核打击后进行核反击。(改自：参考文献[34])	**self-defensive nuclear counterattack** Nuclear counterattack launched after absorbing an opponent's first nuclear attack. (Modified from: Reference [34])
自愿提交协定【zìyuàn tíjiāo xiédìng】	**voluntary offer agreement**
综合国力【zōnghé guólì】	**comprehensive national power**
钻探取样【zuāntàn qǔyàng】	**drilling to obtain radioactive samples**
最大核威慑【zuìdà héwēishè】 部分中国军事学者以前描述一种核威慑形式所使用的术语，即用强大的核优势为后盾，以大规模使用核武器作威胁来威慑对手。(改自：参考文献[18]，p359) 参见“**威慑**”	**maximum deterrence** A term used in the past by some Chinese military scholars to describe a form of deterrence whereby with strong nuclear superiority as support, the threat of a massive nuclear strike is used to deter the adversary. (Modified from: Reference [18], p359) Refer to “**deterrence**”

最低核威慑【zuìdī héwēishè】 通过威胁使用最少数量的核武器，产生能够慑止对方攻击所需的最低限度的破坏。(源自：参考文献[24]，p2)	**minimum deterrence** Threatening the lowest level of damage necessary to prevent attack, with the fewest number of nuclear weapons possible. (From: Reference [24], p2)

缩略语

ABM Treaty	**Treaty Between the United States of America and the Union of Soviet Republics on the Limitation of Anti-ballistic Missile Systems**	美苏关于限制反弹道导弹系统条约(反导条约)
AF&F	**Arming, Fuzing & Firing system**	引控系统
ASC Program	**Advanced Simulation and Computing Program**	先进模拟与计算计划
ASCI	**Accelerated Strategic Computing Initiative**	加速战略计算倡议
ASEAN	**Association of Southeast Asian Nations**	东盟
BWR	**Boiling Water Reactor**	沸水堆
C3I	**Command, Control, Communication & Intelligence**	指挥、控制、通信和情报系统(C3I 系统)
C4I	**Command, Control, Communications, Computing & Intelligence**	指挥、控制、通信、计算和情报系统(C4I 系统)
CCD	**Conference of the Committee on Disarmament**	裁军委员会会议
CD	**Conference on Disarmament**	裁军谈判会议
CEP	**Circular Error Probable**	圆概率偏差
CORRTEX	**Continuous Reflectometry for Radius vs Time Experiment**	科尔太克斯法
CSA	**Canned Subassembly**	罐装组件
CSA	**Comprehensive Safeguards Agreement**	全面保障监督协定

CSBMs	Confidence and Security Building Measures	建立信任与安全措施
CTBT	Comprehensive Test Ban Treaty	全面禁止核试验条约
DA	Destructive Analysis	破坏性分析
DIV	Design Information Verification	设计资料核查
DUPIC	Direct Use of Spent PWR Fuel in CANDU Reactors Process	杜皮克工艺
EEL	Essential Equipment List	重要设备清单
ELINT	electronic intelligence	电子情报
ENCD	Eighteen-Nation Committee on Disarmament	十八国裁军委员会
HEU	High-Enriched Uranium	高浓铀
HTGR	High Temperature Gas-Cooled Reactor	高温气冷堆
HWR	Heavy Water Reactor	重水堆
IAEA	International Atomic Energy Agency	国际原子能机构
ICF	Inertial Confinement Fusion	惯性约束聚变
IDC	International Data Center	国际数据中心
IMO	International Maritime Organization	国际海事组织
IMS	International Monitoring System	国际监测系统
INF Treaty	Treaty Between the United States of America and the Union of Soviet Socialist Republics on the Elimination of Their Intermediate-Range and Shorter-Range Missiles	美苏关于消除两国中程及中短程导弹条约(中导条约)
INFCIRC	Information Circular	信息通报

IW	**Information Warfare**	信息战
KMP	**Key Measurement Point**	关键测量点
LEU	**Low-Enriched Uranium**	低浓铀
LOF	**Location Outside Facilities**	设施外场所
LOW	**Launch-on-Warning**	预警即发射
LUA	**Launch-under-Attack**	遇袭即发射
LWR	**Light Water Reactor**	轻水堆
MAD	**Mutual Assured Destruction**	相互确保摧毁
MaRV	**Maneuverable Reentry Vehicle**	机动再入弹头
MBA	**Material Balance Area**	核材料平衡区
MBP	**Material Balance Period**	材料平衡周期
MIRV	**Multiple Independently Targetable Reentry Vehicle**	分导式多弹头
MNSR	**Miniature Neutron Source Reactor**	微型中子源反应堆
MOX	**Mixed Oxide**	混合氧化物
MTCR	**Missile Technology Control Regime**	导弹技术控制制度
MUF	**Material Unaccounted For**	不明材料量
NEM	**Nuclear-Explosive Material**	核爆材料
NEMP	**Nuclear Electromagnetic Pulse**	核电磁脉冲
NIF	**National Ignition Facility**	国家点火装置
NNWS	**Non-Nuclear Weapon State**	无核武器国家
NPT	**Treaty on the Non-Proliferation of Nuclear Weapons**	不扩散核武器条约

NSG	Nuclear Suppliers Group	核供应国集团
NTMs	National Technical Means	国家技术手段
NTS	Nuclear Threshold State	核门槛国家
NWS	Nuclear Weapon State	核武器国家
OSCE	Organization for Security and Cooperation in Europe	欧洲安全与合作组织
OSI	on-site inspection	现场视察
PAL	Permissive Action Link	密码锁(亦称启动连接装置)
PNE	Treaty Between the United States of America and the Union of Soviet Socialist Republics on Underground Nuclear Explosion for Peaceful Purposes	美苏和平利用地下核爆炸条约
PTBT	Treaty Banning Nuclear Weapon Tests in the Atmosphere, in Outer Space and Under Water	禁止在大气层、外层空间和水下进行核武器试验条约
PUREX Process	Plutonium Uranium Recovery by Extraction Process	普雷克斯流程
PWR	Pressurized Water Reactor	压水堆
RDD	Radioactive Dispersal Device	放射性物质散布装置
RMA	Revolution in Military Affairs	军事变革
RRRW	Reduced Residual Radioactivity Weapon	弱剩余放射性武器(3R 弹)
RSAC	Regional System of Accounting for and Control of Nuclear Material	地区核材料衡算和控制系统

SALT II Treaty	**Treaty Between the United States of America and the Union of Soviet Socialist Republics on the Limitation of Strategic Offensive Arms**	美苏限制进攻性战略武器条约
SALT I	**Interim Agreement Between the United States of America and the Union of Soviet Socialist Republics on Certain Measures with Respect to the Limitation of Strategic Offensive Arms**	美苏限制进攻性战略武器的某些措施的临时协定
SAR	**Synthetic Aperture Radar**	合成孔径雷达
SDI	**Strategic Defense Initiative**	战略防御倡议
SORT	**Treaty Between the United States of American and the Russian Federation On Strategic Offensive Reductions**	美俄削减进攻性战略武器条约(莫斯科条约)
SQ	**Significant Quantity**	重要量
SQP	**Small Quantities Protocol**	小数量议定书
SRD	**Shipper/Receiver Difference**	发方/收方差额
SSAC	**State System of Accounting for and Control of Nuclear Material**	国家核材料衡算和控制系统
START I	**Treaty Between the United States of America and the Union of Soviet Socialist Republics on the Reduction and Limitation of Offensive Strategic Arms**	美苏关于削减和限制进攻性战略武器条约
START II	**Treaty Between the United States of America and the Russian Federation on Further Reduction and Limitation of Strategic Offensive Arms**	美俄关于进一步削减和限制进攻性战略武器条约
THOREX Process	**Thorium Extraction Process**	梭雷克斯流程

TNCD	**Ten-Nation Committee on Disarmament**	十国裁军委员会
TTBT	**Treaty Between the United States of America and the Union of Soviet Socialist Republics on the Limitation of Underground Nuclear Weapon Tests**	美苏限制地下核武器试验条约(限当量条约)
UNDC	**United Nations Disarmament Commission**	联合国裁军审议委员会
UNIDIR	**United Nations Institute for Disarmament Research**	联合国裁军研究所
V&V	**verification and validation**	验证与确认

参考文献

[1] 刘华秋 主编. 军备控制与裁军手册[M]. 北京: 国防工业出版社, 2000.
Liu Huaqiu. Arms Control and Disarmament Handbook. Beijing: National Defense Industry Press, 2000.

[2] 国防科技名词大典——核能卷编委会. 国防科技名词大典——核能[M]. 北京: 航空工业出版社, 兵器工业出版社, 原子能出版社, 2002.
Edit Committee of National Defense Science and Technology Dictionary－Nuclear Energy Column. National Defense Science and Technology Dictionary－Nuclear Energy. Beijing: Aviation Industry Press, Enginery Industry Press, Atomic Energy Press, 2002.

[3] 中国军事百科全书编审委员会. 中国军事百科全书(第 5, 6 卷)[M]. 北京: 军事科学出版社, 1997.
Edit Committee for Chinese Military Encyclopedia. Chinese Military Encyclopedia (Volume 5, 6). Beijing: Military Science Press, 1997.

[4] 国际原子能机构(IAEA). 国际原子能机构保障监督术语[M/OL]//国际核查丛书 (2001 版)[M]. 维也纳: IAEA, 2002.
International Atomic Energy Agency (IAEA). IAEA Safeguards Glossary 2001 Edition. International Nuclear Verification Series No.3. Vienna: IAEA, 2002. Available as of March 2008 at:
http://www-pub.iaea.org/MTCD/publications/PDF/nvs-3-cd/PDF/NVS3_scr.pdf

[5] 北大西洋公约组织(NATO). 北约英俄核术语词典[M/OL]. 北约, 2007.
North Atlantic Treaty Organization. NATO English and Russian Nuclear Terms. NATO, 2007. Available as of March 2008 at:
http://www.nato.int/docu/glossary/eng-nuclear/nuc_glos-e.pdf

[6] Shelkh Ali. 和平与核战争词典[M]. Santa Barbara, CA: ABC-Clio 信息部, 1989.
Sheikh Ali. The Peace and Nuclear War Dictionary. Santa Barbara, CA: ABC-Clio Information Services, 1989.

[7] 国家科学院国际安全和军控委员会(CISAC). 美国未来核武器政策[M/OL]. 华盛顿特区: 国家科学院出版社, 1997.
Committee on International Security and Arms Control (CISAC) of the National Academy of Sciences. The Future of U.S. Nuclear Weapons Policy, Washington, D.C.: The National Academies Press, 1997. Available as of March 2008 at: http://www.nap.edu/catalog.php?record_id=5796

[8] 美国国务院. 军控与裁军术语表[M/OL].
U.S. Department of State: Arms Control and Disarmament Glossary of Terms. Available as of March 2008 at:
http://usinfo.state.gov/is/Archive_Index/Arms_Control_and_Disarmament_Glossary_of_Terms.html

[9] 美国国防部, 参谋长联席会议. 国防部军事及相关术语词典[M/OL]. 2007.
Department of Defense, Joint Chiefs of Staff. Department of Defense Dictionary of Military and Associated Terms, 1-02. 2007. Available as of March 2008 at:
http://www.dtic.mil/doctrine/jel/new_pubs/jp1_02.pdf or
http://www.dtic.mil/doctrine/jel/doddict

[10] Rene Bierbaum 等. 能源部核武器可靠性定义: 历史, 描述和执行[R/OL]. 圣地亚国家实验室, SAND99-8240 报告, 1999.
Rene Bierbaum, et al. DOE Nuclear Weapon Reliability Definition: History, Description, and Implementation. Sandia National Laboratories, report SAND99-8240, 1999. Available as of March 2008 at:
http://www.osti.gov/bridge/purl.cover.jsp?purl=/6105-eS62Sb/webviewable/ or
http://www.osti.gov/bridge/servlets/purl/6105-eS62Sb/webviewable/6105.PDF

[11] 国家科学院国际安全和军控委员会(CISAC). 监察核武器及核爆材料: 方法与能力评估[R/OL]. 华盛顿特区: 国家学院出版社, 2005.
Committee on International Security and Arms Control (CISAC) of the National Academy of Sciences. Monitoring Nuclear Weapons and Nuclear-Explosive Materials: An Assessment of Methods and Capabilities. Washington, D.C.: The National Academies Press, 2005. Available as of March 2008 at:
http://www.nap.edu/catalog.php?record_id=11265

[12] 科学与国际安全研究所 (ISIS) . ISIS 非法采购网络的案例研究, 电子书术语[M/OL]. 2003.
Institute for Science and International Security (ISIS). ISIS Case Studies of Illicit Procurement Networks, E-Book Glossary, 2003. Available as of March 2008 at: http://www.exportcontrols.org/glossary.html

[13] 国家科学院国际安全和军控委员会(CISAC). 管理和控制剩余的武器级钚[M/OL]. 华盛顿特区: 国家学院出版社, 1994.
Committee on International Security and Arms Control (CISAC) of the National Academy of Sciences. The Management and Disposition of Excess Weapons

参考
文献

Plutonium. Washington D.C.: The National Academies Press, 1994. Available as of March 2008 at: http://www.nap.edu/catalog.php?record_id=2345

[14] 国际原子能机构(IAEA). 国家核燃料循环概况[M/OL]. 技术报告序列号 No.404. 维也纳, IAEA, 2001.

International Atomic Energy Agency (IAEA). Country Nuclear Fuel Cycle Profiles. Technical Reports Series No.404, Vienna: IAEA, 2001. Available as of March 2008 at:
http://www-pub.iaea.org/MTCD/publications/PDF/TRS404_scr.pdf

[15] 国际原子能机构(IAEA). 国际原子能机构与《不扩散核武器条约》有关国家之间协议的框架和内容. INFIRCIR/153 协议, 奥地利: IAEA, 1972.

International Atomic Energy Agency (IAEA).The Structure and Content of Agreements Between the Agency and States Required in Connection with the Treaty on the Non-Proliferation of Nuclear Weapons. IAEA INFCIRC/153. Austria: IAEA, 1972. Available as of March 2008 at:
http://www.iaea.org/Publications/Documents/Infcircs/Others/infcirc153.pdf

[16] 联合国裁军研究所(裁研所)和核查、研究、培训和信息中心(核查). 安全术语: 核查与遵约手册[M]. 瑞士・日内瓦: 联合国裁军研究所(UNIDIR); 英国・伦敦: 核查研究、培训和信息中心(VERTIC). UNDIR/2003/10.

United Nations Institute for Disarmament Research (UNIDIR) and The Verification Research, Training and Information Centre (VERTIC). Coming to Terms with Security: A Handbook on Verification and Compliance. Geneva, Switzerland and London, United Kingdom: UNIDIR and VERTIC, 2003. UNIDIR/2003/10.

[17] 罗纳德・里根. 关于国家安全的全国讲话[R/OL]. [1983-03-23].

Ronald Reagan. Address to the Nation on National Security. March 23, 1983. Available as of March 2008 at:
http://www.globalsecurity.org/space/library/congress/1996_cr/s960329a.htm

[18] 王文荣. 战略学[M]. 北京: 国防大学出版社, 1999.

Wang Wenrong. Science of Military Strategy. Beijing: National Defense University Press, 1999.

[19] Steven Tulliu, Thomas Schmalberger. 安全术语: 军控、裁军和建立信任措施词典[M/OL]. 日内瓦: 联合国裁军研究所. UNDIR/2003/22.

Steven Tulliu and Thomas Schmalberger. Coming To Terms with Security: A Lexicon for Arms Control, Disarmament and Confidence Building. Geneva:

United Nations Institute for Disarmament Research, 2003. UNDIR/2003/22. Available as of March 2008 at: http://www.unidir.ch/pdf/ouvrages/pdf-1-92-9045-156-4-en.pdf

[20] William Graham 等. 评估电磁脉冲攻击对美国的威胁的委员会报告[R/OL]. 公共法, 2004: 106-398.
William Graham et al. Report of the Commission to Assess the Threat to the United States from Electromagnetic Pulse (EMP) Attack. 2004. Public Law 106-398. Available as of March 2008 at: http://www.globalsecurity.org/wmd/library/congress/2004_r/04-07-22emp.pdf

[21] 美国国防部. 四年一度防务评估[R/OL]. 国防部, 2006.
亦见: Charles Lutes. 威慑能定制吗? 无限制战争讨论会年报[R/OL]. Johns Hopkins 大学应用物理实验室, 2007.
Department of Defense. The Quadrennial Defense Review. Department of Defense, February 2006. Available as of March 2008 at: http://www.defenselink.mil/pubs/pdfs/QDR20060203.pdf.
See also: Charles Lutes. Can Deterrence Be Tailored? Unrestricted Warfare Symposium Proceedings 2007. Johns Hopkins University Applied Physics Laboratory. Available as of March 2008 at: http://www.jhuapl.edu/urw_symposium/previous/2007/pages/proceedings/2007/papers/Lutes.pdf

[22] Keir Lieber , Daryl Press. 美国核优势的升起[J]. 外交事务, 2006, 3 月－4 月.
Keir Lieber and Daryl Press. The Rise of U.S. Nuclear Primacy. Foreign Affairs, March/April 2006. Available as of March 2008 at: http://www.foreignaffairs.org/20060301faessay85204/keir-a-lieber-daryl-g-press/the-rise-of-u-s-nuclear-primacy.html

[23] Thomas Schelling. 军备及影响[M]. New Haven, CT: 耶鲁大学出版社, 1966.
Thomas Schelling. Arms and Influence. New Haven, CT: Yale University Press, 1966.

[24] Peter Gizewski. 世界新秩序中的最低核威慑[C]//极光论文(24). 渥太华: 加拿大全球安全中心, 1994.
Peter Gizewski. Minimum Nuclear Deterrence in a New World Order. Aurora Papers No. 24. Ottawa: Canadian Centre for Global Security, 1994.

[25] 中华人民共和国核出口管制条例 (修订版)[M]. 2001.
Regulations of the People's Republic of China on the Control of Nuclear Export. Revised Edition. 2001.

参考文献

[26] 连培生. 原子能工业(修订版)[M]. 北京: 原子能出版社, 2002.

Lian Peisheng. Atomic Energy Industry (Revised Edition). Beijing: Atomic Energy Press, 2002.

[27] Lynn Eden 和 Steven Miller, eds. 核问题辩论: 对战略核武器与军备控制争论的理解[M]. 纽约: 康奈尔大学出版社, 1989.

Lynn Eden and Steven Miller, eds. Nuclear Arguments: Understanding the Strategic Nuclear Arms and Arms Control Debates. New York: Cornell University Press, 1989.

[28] John Baylis 等. 现代战略Ⅰ: 理论和概念(Phil Williams, "危机管理"部分)[M]. 伦敦和悉尼: Croom Helm 出版社, 1987.

Phil Williams. Crisis Management. In: John Baylis et al. Contemporary Strategy I: Theories and Concepts. London and Sydney: Croom Helm, 1987.

[29] 北大西洋公约组织(NATO). 非北约核术语和定义词汇表[M]//北约－俄罗斯核术语和定义词汇表, 附录 2[M/OL]. NATO, 2007.

North Atlantic Treaty Organization(NATO). NATO-Russia Glossary of Nuclear Terms and Definitions. Appendix 2: Non-NATO Nuclear Terms and Definitions. NATO, 2007. Available as of March 2008 at:
http://www.nato.int/docu/glossary/eng-nuclear/nuc_glos-e.pdf

[30] Robert Thorn, Donald Westervelt. 流体核试验[R], LA-10902-MS UC-2. 洛斯・阿拉莫斯: 洛斯・阿拉莫斯国家实验室, 1987.

Robert Thorn and Donald Westervelt. Hydronuclear Experiments, LA-10902-MS UC-2. Los Alamos: Los Alamos National Laboratory, 1987.

[31] 彭广谦 等著. 战略学[M]. 北京: 军事科学院出版, 2001.

Peng Guangqian et al. Science of Military Strategy. Beijing: Academy of Military Sciences Press, 2001.

[32] Hangbok Choi 等. DUPIC 燃料兼容性分析进展 - I: 反应堆物理[J]. 核技术, 2006,153(1).

Hangbok Choi et al. Progress of the DUPIC Fuel Compatibility Analysis - I: Reactor Physics. Nuclear Technology, 2006, 153 (1).

[33] 王厚卿, 张兴业. 战役学[M]. 北京: 国防大学出版社, 2000.

Wang Houqing, Zhang Xingye. Science of Campaign. Beijing: National Defense University, 2000.

[34] 中华人民共和国. 2006 年中国的国防[M/OL]. 中华人民共和国国务院新闻办公室.

北京. [2006-12].

People's Republic of China. China's National Defense in 2006. Information Office of the State Council of the People's Republic of China. Beijing: December 2006. Available as of March 2008 at: http://www.chinadaily.com.cn/china/2006-12/29/content_771191.htm

[35] 1978年核不扩散法案[M]. 公共法.1978, 95-242.

Nuclear Non-Proliferation Act of 1978, Public Law 95-242. Available as of March 2008 at: http://www.nti.org/db/china/engdocs/nnpa1978.htm

[36] 中国军事网. 中国人手里会没有"杀手锏"吗? [EB/OL].

China Military Net. Could the Chinese be Without "Assassin's Mace" in Hands? Available as of March 2008 at: http://military.china.com/zh_cn/critical3/27/20060216/13099404.html

[37] 洛斯・阿拉莫斯国家实验室. NNSA先进的模拟和计算程序[CP/OL].

Los Alamos National Laboratory. NNSA Advanced Simulation and Computing Program Website. Available as of March 2008 at: http://www.lanl.gov/projects/asci/

[38] 人民网. 中国建立法制化防扩散出口管制体系[EB/OL]. [2003-12-04].

People Net. China's Established Legal Systems for Non-proliferation and Export Controls. December 4, 2003. Available as of March 2008 at: http://www.people.com.cn/GB/junshi/1076/2227410.html

[39] Jamie Ann Calabrese . 胡萝卜还是大棒?利比亚和美国针对无赖国家所做的努力[J/OL]. 战略观察, 2004, 3 (11).

Jamie Ann Calabrese. Carrots or Sticks? Libya and U.S. Efforts to Influence Rogue States. Strategic Insights. Volume 3 (11), 2004. Available as of March 2008 at: https://www.maxwell.af.mil/au/awc/awcgate/nps/ccc_calabrese_nov04.pdf

[40] 美国国务院. 凯南及围堵政策[M/OL]. 1947.

U.S. Department of State. Kennan and Containment, 1947. Available as of March 2008 at: http://www.state.gov/r/pa/ho/time/cwr/17601.htm

[41] David Yost. 劝阻和盟国[J/OL]. 战略观察, 2005, 4 (2).

David Yost. Dissuasion and Allies. Strategic Insights. 2005, 4 (2). Available as of March 2008 at: http://www.ccc.nps.navy.mil/si/2005/Feb/yostfeb05.asp

[42] 美国国务院. 八国集团.

U.S. Department of State. The G-8 Global Partnership. Available as of March 2008 at: http://www.state.gov/t/isn/c12743.htm

[43] 2006 俄罗斯联邦任期八国集团官方网站. 八国集团历史.
Official Website of the G-8 Presidency of the Russian Federation in 2006. G-8 History. Available as of March 2008 at: http://en.g8russia.ru/g8/history/shortinfo/

[44] 情况说明书: 对核恐怖主义作战的全球计划.
The Global Initiative to Combat Nuclear Terrorism. Fact Sheet. Available as of March 2008 at: http://www.whitehouse.gov/news/releases/2006/07/print/20060715-3.html

[45] Sara Wood. 有官员称，平衡对中美关系至关重要. 美国军方新闻部. [2006-03-17].
Sara Wood. Balance Critical to U.S.-China Relationship, Officials Say. American Forces Press Service, March 17, 2006. Available as of March 2008 at: http://www.defenselink.mil/news/newsarticle.aspx?id=15136

[46] Alastair Iain Johnston. 中国新的"旧思维" [J]. 国际安全, 1995/1996, 20(3).
Alastair Iain Johnston. China's New "Old Thinking". International Security, 1995/96, 20 (3).

[47] 核供应集团(NSG)网站.
The Nuclear Suppliers Group (NSG) Website. Available as of March 2008 at: http://www.nuclearsuppliersgroup.org/

[48] 美国国会图书馆, 联邦政府研究部. 苏联术语表[M]//国家研究地域手册丛书[M/OL].
Library of Congress. Federal Research Division, Countries Studies Area Handbook Series, Glossary - Soviet Union. Available as of March 2008 at: http://lcweb2.loc.gov/frd/cs/soviet_union/su_glos.html

[49] 北大西洋公约组织(NATO). 北约和北约－俄罗斯核术语和定义[M] //北约－俄罗斯核术语和定义词汇表, 附录 1[M/OL]. NATO, 2007.
North Atlantic Treaty Organization. NATO-Russia Glossary of Nuclear Terms and Definitions. Appendix 1: NATO and NATO-Russia Nuclear Terms and Definitions. NATO, 2007. Available as of March 2008 at: http://www.nato.int/docu/glossary/eng-nuclear/

[50] 美国国防部. 美国国防部合作减少威胁(CTR)计划网站[EB/OL]. 1998.
Department of Defense. Department of Defense Cooperative Threat Reduction (CTR) Program Website,1998. Available as of March 2008 at:

http://www.dod.mil/pubs/ctr/instability.html

[51] 国际原子能机构(IAEA). IAEA 保障监督: 防止核武器扩散[EB/OL]. 新闻通告. 2002.

International Atomic Energy Agency (IAEA). IAEA Safeguards: Stemming the Spread of Nuclear Weapons. Factsheet. 2002. Available as of March 2008 at: http://www.iaea.org/Publications/Factsheets/English/S1_Safeguards.pdf

[52] 新华网. 核材料实物保护公约: 加强对核设施核材料保护[EB/OL]. [2005-07-08].

Xinhua Net. Convention on the Physical Protection of Nuclear Material: Enhancing Physical Protection of Nuclear Material and Facilities. Xinhua Net. July 8, 2005. Available as of March 2008 at: http://news.xinhuanet.com/world/2005-07/09/content_3195596.htm

[53] 中华人民共和国驻印度大使. 记者招待会: 和平共处五项基本原则. 和平共处五项基本原则提出 50 周年纪念[EB/OL]. [2004-06-14].

Embassy of the People's Republic of China in India. Backgrounder: Five Principles of Peaceful Coexistence. The 50th Anniversary of the Initiation of the Five Principles of Peaceful Co-Existence. June 14 2004. Available as of March 2008 at: http://in.china-embassy.org/eng/ssygd/fiveprinciple/t132640.htm

[54] 联合国裁军研究所(裁研所)和核查、研究、培训和信息中心(核查). 关键术语[M]// 安全术语: 核查与遵约手册[M/OL]. 瑞士日内瓦和英国伦敦: UNIDIR 和 VERTIC. 2003.

United Nations Institute for Disarmament Research (UNIDIR) and The Verification Research, Training and Information Centre (VERTIC). Coming to Terms with Security: A Handbook on Verification and Compliance. Key Terms. Geneva, Switzerland and London, United Kingdom: UNIDIR and VERTIC, 2003. Available as of March 2008 at: http://www.unidir.org/pdf/articles/pdf-art1980.pdf

[55] Steven Lambakis. 重新审议非对称战争[J]. 联合军力季刊, 2005, (36).

Steven Lambakis. Reconsidering Asymmetric Warfare. Joint Force Quarterly, 2005, (36). Available as of March 2008 at: http://www.dtic.mil/doctrine/jel/jfq_pubs/1736.pdf

[56] Michael Krepon, Christopher Clary. 确保外空还是统治外空? 反对外空武器化的案例[M]. 华盛顿特区: Henry L. Stimson 中心, 2003.

Michael Krepon with Christopher Clary. Space Assurance or Space Dominance? The Case Against Weaponizing Space. Washington, D.C.: The Henry L.

参考文献

Stimson Center, 2003. Available as of March 2008 at:
http://www.stimson.org/wos/pdf/space2.pdf

[57] Celeste Wallander. 得与失: 戈尔巴乔夫的"新思维"[J]. 华盛顿季刊, 2002, 25(1).
Celeste Wallander. Lost and Found: Gorbachev's "New Thinking". The Washington Quarterly, 2002, 25 (1). Available as of March 2008 at:
http://www.twq.com/02winter/wallander.pdf

[58] Matthew Evangelista. 非武装力量: 结束冷战的跨国努力[M]. 纽约伊萨卡: 康内尔大学出版社, 1999.
Matthew Evangelista. Unarmed Forces: The Transnational Effort to End the Cold War. Ithaca, N.Y.: Cornell University Press, 1999.

[59] 国家科学院国际安全和军控委员会(CISAC). 有关"全面禁止核试验条约" 批准的技术问题[M/OL]. 华盛顿特区: 国家学院出版社, 2002.
Committee on International Security and Arms Control (CISAC) of the National Academy of Sciences. Technical Issues Related to Ratification of the Comprehensive Nuclear Test Ban Treaty. Washington, D.C.: The National Academies Press, 2002. Available as of March 2008 at:
http://www.nap.edu/catalog.php?record_id=10471

[60] 美国国防部部长副助理核问题办公室. 核武器确信性.
Office to the Deputy Assistant to the Secretary of Defense for Nuclear Matters. Nuclear Weapons Surety. Available as of March 2008 at:
http://www.acq.osd.mil/ncbdp/nm/nuclearweaponssurety.html

[61] 美国陆军司令部. 战场手册(No.1)[M/OL]. 华盛顿特区: 陆军部, 2005.
U.S. Department of the Army. Field Manual No.1. Washington D.C.: Department of the Army, 2005. Available as of March 2008 at:
http://www.army.mil/fm1/chapter3.html

[62] Albert Latter, Ernest Martinelli. 主动和被动防御[EB/OL]. 1965.
Albert Latter and Ernest Martinelli. Active and Passive Defense, 1965. Available as of March 2008 at:
http://stinet.dtic.mil/cgi-bin/GetTRDoc?AD=AD676973&Location=U2&doc=GetTRDoc.pdf

[63] Martin Pilch 等. 圣地亚 ASCI 验证与确认计划的指导方针－内容与形式: 版本 2.0[R/OL]. SAND2000-3101, 非限制发行, 2001.
Martin Pilch, et al. Guidelines for Sandia ASCI Verification and Validation Plans

参考文献

- Content and Format: Version 2.0. SAND2000-3101, Unlimited Distribution, 2001. Available as of March 2008 at: http://www.prod.sandia.gov/cgi-bin/techlib/access-control.pl/2000/003101.pdf

[64] 戈尔巴乔夫. 诺贝尔演讲[R/OL]. [1991-06-05].
Mikhail Gorbachev. Nobel Lecture. June 5, 1991. Available as of March 2008 at: http://nobelprize.org/nobel_prizes/peace/laureates/1990/gorbachev-lecture.html

参考文献

[65] Gareth Evans. 第 48 界联合国大会第五次全体会议上的讲话[R/OL]. [1993-9-27].
Gareth Evans. Speech to the 5th Plenary Meeting of the 48th Session of the United Nations General Assembly. September 27, 1993. Available as of March 2008 at:
http://www.crisisgroup.org/library/documents/speeches_ge/foreign_minister/1993/270993_fm_uncooperatingforpeaces.pdf

[66] Douglas Feith. 国防部副部长 Douglas J. Feith 关于政策的讲话[C]//参议院军事事务听证会听取《核态势评估》报告[R/OL]. [2002-02-14].
Douglas Feith. Statement of the Honorable Douglas J. Feith, Undersecretary of Defense for Policy, Senate Armed Services Hearing on the Nuclear Posture Review. February 14, 2002. Available as of March 2008 at:
http://armed-services.senate.gov/statement/2002/Feith.pdf

[67] 美国国防部. 美国核态势评估(摘录)[R]. 2001 年 12 月 31 日递交. 美国国防部, [2002-01-08].
Department of Defense. U.S. Nuclear Posture Review (Excerpts). Submitted to Congress on December 31, 2001. Department of Defense. January 8, 2002. Available as of March 2008 at:
http://www.globalsecurity.org/wmd/library/policy/dod/npr.htm.

[68] Linton Brooks. Linton F. Brooks 大使(美国能源部副部长、国家核安全管理局局长)在众议院武装力量委员会战略力量分委会上的陈述[R/OL]. [2006-03-01].
Linton Brooks. Statement of Ambassador Linton F. Brooks, Under Secretary for Nuclear Security and Administrator, National Nuclear Security Administration U.S. Department of Energy Before the House Armed Services Committee Subcommittee on Strategic Forces. March 1, 2006. Available as of March 2008 at:
http://www.nipp.org/Adobe/RRW%20final%20with%20foreword%207.30.07.pdf

[69] Gregory Giles 等. 最低核威慑研究：最终报告[R/OL]. 国防部减小威胁局先进系

统与概念办公室. [2003-05-15].

Gregory Giles et al. Minimum Nuclear Deterrence Research: Final Report. Advanced Systems and Concepts Office, Defense Threat Reduction Agency. May 15, 2003. Available as of March 2008 at: http://www.dtra.mil/documents/asco/publications/MinimumNuclearDeterrencePhase2.pdf

[70] 王仲春. 核武器核国家核战略[M]. 北京: 时事出版社, 2007.

Wang Zhongchun. Nuclear Weapons, Nuclear States, Nuclear Strategy. Beijing: Current Events Publishing House, 2007.

[71] 美国技术评估办公室. 威慑、美国核战略和弹道导弹防御[J]. 弹道导弹防御技术, 1985.

U.S. Office of Technology Assessment. Deterrence, U.S. Nuclear Strategy, and BMD. Ballistic Missile Defense Technologies. 1985. Available as of March 2008 at: http://www.princeton.edu/~ota/disk2/1985/8504/8504.PDF

[72] James Russell, James Wirtz. 静悄悄的变革: 新的核三位一体[J/OL]. 战略观察, 2002, 1 (3).

James Russell and James Wirtz. A Quiet Revolution: The New Nuclear Triad. Strategic Insights. 2002,1(3). Available as of March 2008 at: http://www.ccc.nps.navy.mil/si/may02/triad.asp

[73] 中华人民共和国国务院. 中华人民共和国核两用品及相关技术出口管制条例(修订版)[M/OL]. [2007-01-26].

The State Council of the People's Republic of China. Regulations of the People's Republic of China on Export Control of Dual-Use Nuclear Goods and the Related Technologies. Revised Edition. January 26, 2007. Available as of March 2008 at:
http://www.gov.cn/zwgk/2007-02/16/content_529172.htm

[74] 中华人民共和国国务院. 中华人民共和国核出口管制条例(修订版)[M/OL]. [2006-11-09]The State Council of the People's Republic of China. Regulations of the People's Republic of China on the Control of Nuclear Export. Revised Edition. November 9, 2006. Available as of March 2008 at:
http://www.gov.cn/zwgk/2006-12/01/content_459513.htm

参考文献